TRAINING

INTERNATIONAL DAN

AF700911

• DAN America •

Director of Training — William Clendenen
Training Staff Specialist — Kimberley Walker
Training Staff Specialist — David Lawler

• DAN Japan •

Director of Medicine — Yoshihiro Mano, M.D.
Director General — Masaki Hayano
Training Specialist — Tetsu Nozawa

• DAN Southeast Asia-Pacific •

Executive Director & Training Director — John Lippmann

• DAN Southern Africa •

Executive Director — Frans Cronjé, M.D.

• DAN Europe •

President — Alessandro Marroni, M.D.
Vice President Training & Education — Ulrich van Laak, M.D.

European Regional Offices

Benelux — Costantino Balestra, Ph.D.
Croatia — Darko Kovacevic, M.D.
Deutschland/Austria — Ulrich van Laak, M.D.
Iberica — Jordi Desola, M.D.
Italia — Nuccia De Angelis, Ph.D.
Malta — Ramiro Cali Corleo, M.D.
Skandinavien — Ole Hyldegaard, M.D.
Slovenia — Igor Mekjavic, M.D.
Suisse — Jürg Wendling, M.D.
United Kingdom — Chris Young, Cert. Ed.

DAN America The Peter B. Bennett Center, 6 West Colony Place, Durham, NC 27705 USA
Tel: +1-919-684-2948, 1-800-446-2671
Fax: +1-919-490-6630
www.DiversAlertNetwork.org

DAN America-Mexico c/o Servicio de Medicina Hiperbarica, Hospital Angeles del Pedregal, Camino a Santa Teresa 1055, Heroes de Padierna, C.P. 10700, Mexico D.F., Mexico
Tel: +52-5-568-8082, fax: +52-5-568-8083
danmex@planet.com.mx
www.scubalatin.com.mx/dan/dan.htm

DAN Europe P.O Box DAN, 64026 Roseto (Te), Italy
Tel: +39-085-893-0333
fax: +39-085-893-0050
mail@daneurope.org
www.daneurope.org/main.htm

DAN Japan Japan Marine Recreation Association, 3-8 Mejiro, 1-Chome, Toshima-ku, Tokyo 171-0031, Japan
Tel: +81-3-3590-6501
Fax: +81-3-3590-8325
dan@danjapan.gr.jp
website: www.danjapan.gr.jp

DAN South East Asia-Pacific P.O. Box 384, Ashburton, Victoria 3147, Australia
Tel: +61-3-9886-9166
Fax: +61-3-9886-9155
danseap@danseap.com.au
www.danseap.com.au

DAN Southern Africa P.O. Box 710, Auckland Park 2006 South Africa
Tel: +27-11-242-0380
Fax: +27-11-242-0385
mail@dansa.org
www.dansa.org

International DAN Mission Statement

International Divers Alert Network (IDAN), a non-profit organization, exists to provide expert information and advice consistent with the current medical literature for the benefit of the diving public.

DAN's historical and primary function is to provide emergency medical advice and assistance for underwater diving injuries, to work to prevent injuries and to promote diving safety.

DAN promotes and supports underwater diving research and education, particularly as it relates to the improvement of diving safety, first aid and medical treatment.

DAN strives to provide accurate, up-to-date and unbiased information on issues of common concern to the diving public, and to advocate for divers' concerns, primarily, but not exclusively, for diving safety.

DAN Oxygen First for Scuba Diving Injuries, 4th Edition
Editor: William Clendenen
Principal Authors: Jeffrey J. Bertsch, Dan Orr
Contributors: James Corry, Joel Dovenbarger, John Lippmann, Yoshihiro Mano, M.D., Alessandro Marroni, M.D., G. Yancey Mebane, M.D., Randy Sitzes, Larry "Harris" Taylor, Chris Wachholz, Kimberley Walker

Layout by Leigh Goodwin and Renée Westerfield
Cover Design by Phillip Daquila
Cover Photos by Steve Barnett
Studio Photos by Duke University Medical Center Photographic Services
Photo subjects: Laura S. Clendenen, William Clendenen, Greg Moore
Illustrations by Lisa Sparks

Fourth Edition published February 1997
— ISBN 0-9656942-0-8
Third edition published November 1994
Second edition published April 1994
First edition published November 1993

INTERNATIONAL DAN

A Message from Dr. Peter Bennett

This workbook is dedicated to divers around the world in pursuit of one of the important missions of International DAN (IDAN): its intent is to assure that, in the event of a diving injury resulting in decompression illness, oxygen and individuals trained in its use are available at every dive site and on every dive boat.

After the ABCs (assuring Airway, Breathing and Circulation), the delivery of 100 percent oxygen as soon as possible is now widely recognized as critical first aid for diving injuries such as decompression sickness (DCS), arterial gas embolism and near-drowning. Yet, recent DAN America data (based on 1995 information) shows that only 37 percent of injured divers actually receive oxygen. Internationally, the incidence of providing oxygen is probably even lower.

I am reminded of an incident on a Pacific island that occurred on one of DAN's diving physiology and medicine training courses for physicians. We had taken oxygen for the boats with us since the boats provided none. In fact, an arterial gas embolism (AGE) or near-drowning occurred in front of our boat. On retrieving the unresponsive diver, I asked the physicians on board to prepare the oxygen unit. Without proper training, however, they did not know how to assemble it quickly. I had to do the job.

After breathing oxygen for 15 minutes, the injured diver woke up while the boat was returning to shore. Coupled with a subsequent recompression treatment in the hyperbaric chamber, the diver made a complete recovery. But what if we did not have the oxygen unit and there was no trained person to assemble it and give oxygen? Would the diver still have recovered?

Clearly, even training as a physician does not prepare one for assembly of unfamiliar equipment. Thus, one not only needs the right equipment to be able to deliver the correct amount of oxygen, but trained individuals who can assemble the equipment, deliver the oxygen with other necessary first aid, and know how to contact DAN emergency services and get the diver to the nearest emergency department or hyperbaric chamber.

In a diving accident there is significant data to show that delayed treatment can lead to more permanent disability. The role of the delivery of emergency oxygen at the earliest possible moment — which means on the boat or on shore — is also critical in this regard.

You, as a trained oxygen provider, are a vital link in the chain of survival for diving injuries. As DAN grows internationally, we are pleased to be able to offer this student workbook to divers around the world.

over

With a DAN course and this workbook, you will be well prepared and equipped in the event of a dive emergency.

Fundamental to any training program is such a student workbook. This one is written by the DAN Training staff and provides a source of information for students involved in the *Oxygen First Aid for Scuba Diving Injuries* course. It addresses a wide range of topics, including symptom recognition, mechanisms of injury, oxygen equipment and delivery techniques. Even though it is an entry-level course, its comprehensive curriculum will satisfy the interests of the general diving public and the healthcare professional.

The skills you learn in this course will make a significant difference to the outcome of someone with a diving injury. Practice your skills often, and be prepared to provide emergency oxygen first aid with skill and knowledge to your buddy in need. International DAN is proud to be able to help you in this regard and in keeping with our mandate of divers helping divers.

Peter B. Bennett, Ph.D., D.Sc.
President IDAN
Executive Director DAN America

Table of Contents

What is DAN and How Does it Work?

DAN's Diving Emergency Hotline provides a central location for diving emergency coordination, uniting dive physicians and hyperbaric chamber facilities into an international communications network.

Divers Alert Network *(DAN)* is an international, non-profit dive safety organization supported by its members, the largest association of recreational divers in the world. Since 1980, DAN's primary mission has been to improve diving safety for all recreational divers.

DAN accomplishes this goal by providing medical consultation for injured divers, collecting and analyzing diving injury and fatality information, promoting educational training programs, and by offering diving accident insurance and worldwide medical evacuation coverage to its members. In addition, DAN members receive a number of valuable dive and travel benefits.

DAN's efforts are supported by a network of diving medicine professionals, hyperbaric facilities, scuba diving instructors, dive stores, training associations, clubs and dive equipment manufacturers.

Ask your DAN Oxygen Instructor for more information about joining DAN.

DAN Telephone Services

DAN provides two primary phone lines in support of diving safety. All divers, both DAN Members and nonmembers, can call and receive the most current information about diving safety from the DAN Dive Safety and Medical Information Line.

If you suspect you've been injured while diving, you can call DAN's Diving Emergency Hotline. DAN provides this service to the diving community 24 hours a day, 365 days a year to assist and arrange for evaluation and treatment of injured divers by a physician trained in diving medicine. DAN can also help coordinate transportation to the nearest medical facility.

DAN's Hotline: Your Link to Assistance

DAN's Diving Emergency Hotline provides a central location for diving emergency coordination, uniting dive physicians and hyperbaric chamber facilities into an international communications network. DAN handles an increasing number of emergency calls each year.

Most symptoms of decompression illness occur within 24 hours of diving. Sometimes, symptoms are not recognized until the middle of the night. Whenever divers need help, all they have to do is pick up the phone and call DAN or a DAN-supported emergency hotline.

Calling the Hotline

Here is what happens when a diver calls DAN or a DAN-supported Diving Emergency Hotline:

(Note: This procedure can vary from country to country, based on local medical services and protocol.)

1. The call is answered by an operator. After telling the operator that the diver has a diving emergency, the caller will be connected directly with a DAN medical staff member or a physician knowledgeable in diving medicine.

In some instances, it may be necessary for the DAN staff member or physician to return the call at the earliest possible moment.

2. DAN personnel will do one of two things: they will either make an immediate recommendation, or they will return the call after making arrangements with a local physician or the DAN Regional Director/Coordinator.

DAN Regional Directors and Coordinators are familiar with hyperbaric facilities in their area and can make recommendations about treatment.

3. The DAN staff member or Regional Director/Coordinator may ask the caller to wait by the phone while arrangements are being made.

These plans may take up to 30 minutes or longer, as several phone calls may be required for each step.

If it is a life-threatening situation, however, the diver should be transported immediately to the nearest medical facility or emergency department, according to local protocol.

After transport, DAN may be contacted for further consultation. In some very remote diving regions, delays of several hours can occur. While arrangements are being made for evacuation and treatment, the injured diver should receive 100 percent oxygen.

Following *(on Page 8)* is a list of DAN emergency numbers worldwide.

In a life-threatening situation, the diver should be transported immediately to the nearest medical facility or emergency department.

NOTE:
These emergency numbers may change without notice. Ask your DAN Oxygen Instructor or call DAN for the most up-to-date diving emergency contact information.

DAN Diving Emergency Numbers

DAN America . . . . +1-919-684-8111 or
+1-919-684-4DAN (4326) • (-4DAN accepts collect calls)

DAN America-Mexico . . . . +52-5-629-9800 code 9912935
or +52-5-328-2828 code B5100 **or** +52-5-406-0315

DAN Europe . . . . +41-1-1414

DAN Southern Africa
(within South Africa) 0800-020-111
(outside South Africa) . . . . +27-11-242-0112
(+27-11-242-0112 accepts collect calls)

DAN Southeast Asia-Pacific region
Diving Emergency Services (DES)
DES Australia (within Australia) . . 1-800-088-200
DES Australia (from overseas) . . . +61-8-8212-9242
DES New Zealand . . . . +64-9-445-8454
Singapore Naval Medicine
& Hyperbaric Center . . . . +65-750-5546
DAN S.E.A.P.-Philippines . . . . +63-2-815-9911

DAN Medical/Safety Information Line — Your Link to Safety and Health

DAN provides the Dive Safety & Medical Information Line service to help prevent diving injuries.

The DAN Medical/Safety Information Line is operated during normal business hours by medical personnel trained in diving medicine to answer questions about diving medicine, dive safety, fitness for diving, and for providing non-emergency physician referrals. In some regions, these diving information calls are handled by other DAN-supported organizations such as Diving Emergency Services *(DES)* in Australia.

What happens when a diver calls DAN's Dive Safety & Medical Information Line:

1. The caller will be transferred to a specialist trained in diving physiology and medicine. Most of the time, the specialist can answer your questions immediately.

2. If research is required before answering your questions, the specialist will return your call with an answer. In cases where the question refers specifically to a particular diver *(or diving candidate)*, the inquiry may result in a referral to a physician.

DAN provides this service to help prevent diving accidents. By using this service, the diving community is able to effectively educate divers to help reduce their risk of injury.

If problems do occur following a dive, call the DAN or DAN-supported emergency hotline in your area to help determine the most appropriate course of action.

DAN Oxygen First Aid for Diving Injuries

DAN *Oxygen First Aid for Scuba Diving Injuries* course represents entry-level training designed to educate divers and interested nondivers *(such as a charter boat captain)* to recognize scuba diving injuries and to provide emergency oxygen first aid.

Emergency oxygen should be provided for the injured diver while activating the local emergency medical system (EMS) or other similar local procedure and arranging for transportation to the nearest available medical facility.

Education, Training, Recognition & Response

The objective of this course is to educate divers about diving injuries and to train them to use oxygen while providing other assistance. In addition, this course will introduce novice divers to the fundamentals of dive accident recognition, response and management. This program provides an excellent training opportunity for divers and continuing education for leadership-level divers and instructors.

Since Oxygen Provider skills deteriorate with time, DAN Training encourages retraining every two years as a minimum following successful completion of the course. DAN Oxygen Providers are trained to provide emergency oxygen as adjunctive first aid to injured divers while awaiting arrival of emergency medical services or evacuation to the nearest available medical facility.

In addition, divers are encouraged to practice these and other diving skills regularly.

All skills performed in an emergency should be within the scope of your training and experience.

For diving leadership and medical personnel, this course is approved for various continuing education requirements.

Contact the DAN Training Department in your region for continuing education course requirements and specifics.

The objective of this course is to educate divers about diving injuries and to train them to use oxygen while providing other assistance.

Emergency oxygen first aid should not be used in lieu of evaluation and definitive care provided by qualified healthcare professionals.

*The DAN Oxygen Provider course does **not** provide training for:*

- Cardiopulmonary resuscitation (CPR)
- Scuba diving rescue and comprehensive dive accident management
- The use of oxygen in non-diving emergencies

DAN Oxygen Provider Course Overview

CPR training is recommended prior to entering the DAN Oxygen Provider course.

This course consists of specific sections, including:

Knowledge Development

Oxygen Provider Skills Development

1) Scene Safety Assessment

2) Rescue Breathing Practice
(also called Expired Air Resuscitation or Artificial Ventilation)

3) Oxygen Equipment Identification

4) Injured Diver Scenarios —

Breathing Injured Diver

Responsive
- demand valve with mask

Unresponsive
- demand valve with mask
- non-rebreather mask

Non-Breathing-to-Breathing Injured Diver

Unresponsive to Responsive
- pocket mask
- demand valve with mask
- non-rebreather mask

Two Injured Divers

Responsive and Unresponsive
- pocket mask
- demand valve with mask
- non-rebreather mask

5) Equipment Familiarization

6) Equipment Disassembly and Reassembly

7) Examination and Review

Course Prerequisites

The recommended minimum age for participation in this course is 12 years. DAN suggests that those with junior diver certification participate in oxygen first aid training with their adult buddy. Some countries, states and local municipalities have minimum age stipulations for the use of emergency oxygen. Age prerequisites may vary from region to region due to local laws about oxygen and its use.

Cardiopulmonary *(CPR)* training from a recognized agency is recommended prior to entering this course.
In some areas, current CPR certification may be required by the Oxygen Instructor as a prerequisite to the course.

Recommended Time Requirements

Classroom *(cognitive)* hours = 1
Practical *(skills)* hours = 3
Course length may vary due to the number of participants, oxygen equipment and mannequins.

Learning Objectives

You must demonstrate familiarity with the signs, symptoms and recognition of dive injuries including decompression illness and near-drowning.

You must be able to demonstrate proper assembly, disassembly and use of all component parts found in the DAN Oxygen Unit, including the multifunction regulator, the demand inhalator valve and mask, non-rebreather mask and pocket mask with supplemental oxygen.

You must successfully complete the DAN Oxygen First Aid for Scuba Diving Injuries examination. Your DAN Oxygen Instructor will review the examination with you to ensure your complete understanding of the material.

As a DAN Oxygen Provider, you must demonstrate familiarity with the signs, symptoms and recognition of dive injuries — decompression illness and near-drowning.

Required Curriculum Subject Areas

You must demonstrate familiarity with each of the following areas:

- **General diving anatomy, physiology & physics**
- **Respiratory system**
- **Cardiovascular system**
- **Recognition of specified diving emergencies**
  - ***DECOMPRESSION ILLNESS (DCI)***
    - ***Decompression Sickness (DCS)***
    - ***Arterial Gas Embolism (AGE)***
  - ***NEAR-DROWNING***
- **Oxygen's effects on the body**
  - ***Benefits and concerns for using oxygen in a dive injury***
- **Emergency oxygen delivery equipment**
  - ***Purpose***
  - ***Types***
  - ***Features***
  - ***Function***
  - ***Care & Maintenance***

You must be able to demonstrate proper assembly, disassembly and use of all component parts found in the DAN Oxygen Unit, including the multi-function regulator, the demand inhalator valve and mask, non-rebreather mask and pocket mask with supplemental oxygen.

Skill Performance Objectives

In order to successfully complete DAN's Oxygen Provider course, you must demonstrate the following skills:

- **Assess scene and oxygen provider safety**
- **Deploy and operate the DAN Oxygen Unit**
- **Select and position appropriate oxygen mask**
- **Remove and secure oxygen mask and oxygen unit**
- **Change oxygen washer**
- **Assemble and disassemble oxygen unit**

In addition, you must demonstrate the proper technique in providing emergency oxygen to simulated injured divers by:

Assuring Airway, Breathing and Circulation *(ABCs)*, using

✦ ***Demand inhalator valve and mask***

- Turn on and secure oxygen system
- Attach mask to demand inhalator valve
- Place mask on injured diver's face

or

✦ ***Constant-flow, non-rebreather mask***

- Turn on and secure oxygen system
- Set appropriate flow rate
- Prime mask *(reservoir bag)*
- Adjust mask to fit injured diver
- Adjust flow rate *(15 to 25 lpm)*
- Remove mask
- Turn off cylinder
- Purge oxygen system

or

✦ ***Pocket mask with supplemental oxygen inlet***

- Use for non-breathing divers
- Correct mask positioning for mouth-to-mask rescue breathing
- Attach oxygen tubing to mask and regulator
- Adjust flow rate *(15 lpm)*
- Perform effective mouth-to-mask rescue breathing

DAN Oxygen Unit Components

- Oxygen cylinder and valve
- Multifunction regulator
- T-handle
- Handwheel/wrench
- Pressure gauge
- Oxygen-compatible washer
- Constant-flow controller
- Barbed constant-flow outlet
- Intermediate pressure hose
- Pressure-activated check valve *(In threaded DISS outlet)*
- Demand inhalator valve
- Oronasal mask
- Non-rebreather mask
- Pocket mask with oxygen inlet and one-way valve

DAN Oxygen Providers learn to assemble and disassemble the oxygen equipment.

The Main Parts of the DAN Oxygen Unit

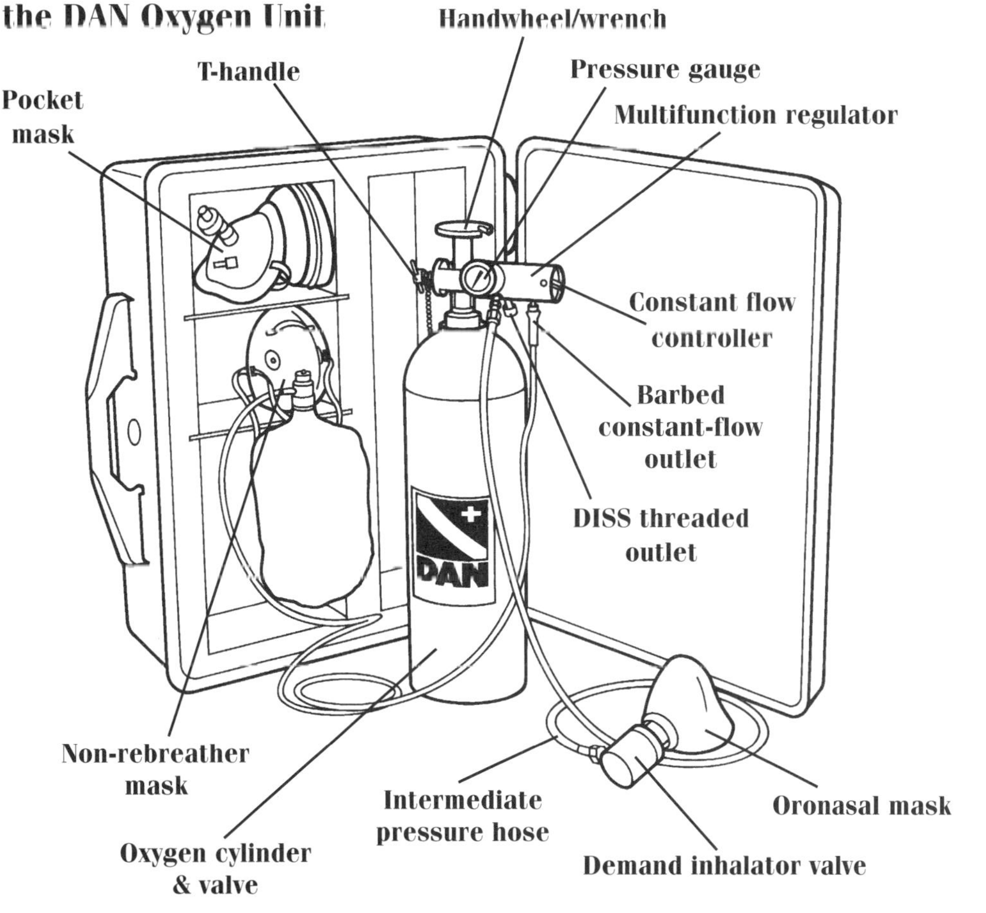

Oxygen First Aid Course Curriculum

OBJECTIVES

In this chapter you'll learn to

1. **Recognize possible dive-related injuries.**
2. **Provide emergency oxygen first aid.**
3. **Activate the local emergency medical system *(EMS)*.**
4. **Arrange transport to the nearest available medical facility.**

Introduction

This workbook provides a guide for oxygen first aid training in the special situations of decompression illness and near-drowning. *The use of oxygen in other situations will not be covered.*

This workbook is a supplement to the DAN *Oxygen First Aid for Diving Injuries* course as taught by a qualified DAN Oxygen Instructor. Learning the proper and effective use of oxygen and oxygen equipment is not difficult, but it requires comprehensive instruction and carefully guided practice with specialized equipment.

Reading this workbook without instruction and practice will not make you competent to use oxygen in an emergency for injured scuba divers.

This course is specifically designed as entry-level training to educate the general diving *(and interested nondiving)* public to recognize possible dive-related injuries and provide emergency oxygen first aid while activating the local emergency medical system *(EMS)* or other similar local procedure and arranging for transportation to the nearest available medical facility.

NOTE: This course does not provide complete training in accident management unless the course is a module and part of a more comprehensive program.

Cardiopulmonary Resuscitation (CPR)

Primary assessment and assuring the ABCs *(Airway, Breathing and Circulation)* are necessary for basic life support and is your highest priority. Training in CPR by an internationally recognized association is important before participating in this course. CPR training will prepare the participant to understand how to effectively deal with many emergencies. Basic life support can be effectively provided to a person without the use of mechanical devices *(airways, resuscitators)* and can be performed by the trained general public. Successes are numerous.

Scuba Certification

This course is intended to teach scuba divers *(also interested non-divers)* how to provide oxygen to injured divers. Familiarity with diving equipment and diving terminology will make understanding the material easier. However, interested and informed non-divers should have little difficulty with this material. Scuba diving certification is not a prerequisite for this course.

The primary goal of first aid is to establish and/or maintain the life of an injured or ill person until assistance becomes available at the scene.

Terminology

The DAN Oxygen Provider Student Workbook uses very few words or terms which might be considered "medical." However, the discussion of the technical concepts in providing oxygen in this workbook does require the use of precise and appropriate terms that may be unfamiliar to you. Technical terms will be defined as they are introduced. Each section of the workbook defines key terms before the material is presented.

Responsibility

The primary goal of first aid is to establish and/or maintain the life of an injured or ill person until assistance *(generally, the emergency medical services — EMS)* arrives or becomes available at the scene. It is equally important that the rescuer do no further harm to the injured person. Providing oxygen to an injured diver will not cause any harm as long as the scene is safe and the oxygen equipment is functioning properly. This means that you must understand the limitations of your skills and knowledge and not attempt any procedure beyond your ability and the scope of your training.

It is important that the rescuer do no further harm to the injured person.

Continuing Education

Continuing education is encouraged in the form of additional training courses, supervised practice sessions, reading current literature and refresher training.

There are several programs that offer advanced training in oxygen administration and dive accident management beyond the entry level. Your DAN Oxygen Instructor can provide you with information regarding these programs, or you can contact the DAN Training Department in your region.

Anatomy & Physiology as it Relates to Oxygen First Aid

OBJECTIVES

In this chapter you'll learn to

1. **Identify the major structures of the respiratory system.**
2. **Identify the major structures of the circulatory system.**
3. **Define hypoxia.**
4. **Identify the area of the lungs where gas exchange occurs.**
5. **List the primary component gases and percentages of air.**

Note: *All information presented in the following sections is based on the most recent diving medical literature. References in the "Related Reading" section of this workbook are available from your Oxygen Instructor or the DAN Training Department in your region.*

KEY TERMS

Familiarizing yourself with these terms at the beginning of each chapter will help you understand the subject matter more quickly.

Alveoli — Microscopic air sacs in the lungs, where gas exchange occurs with the circulatory system.

Aorta — The largest vessel of the systemic arterial system, from which the main arteries carrying oxygenated blood branch and subdivide into smaller and smaller vessels.

Arteriole — Small artery.

Atrium — Chamber of the heart that provides access to another chamber called the ventricle.

Bronchi — Plural of bronchus which is a division of the trachea.

Capillary — Microscopic blood vessels where the gas exchange takes place between the bloodstream and the tissues or air in the lungs.

Carbon Dioxide — A waste gas produced by the metabolism of oxygen in the body.

Carbon Monoxide — A highly poisonous, odorless, tasteless and colorless gas formed when carbon material burns with restricted access to oxygen. It is toxic by inhalation since it competes with oxygen in binding with the hemoglobin, thereby resulting in diminished availability of oxygen in tissues.

Key Terms — *continued from page 16*

Cilia — Long, slender microscopic hairlike processes extending from cells and capable of rhythmic motion.

Esophagus — Portion of the digestive tract that lies between the back of the throat and stomach.

Fossa Ovalis — Oval depression in the wall of the heart remaining when the foramen ovale closes at birth *(See patent foramen ovale).*

Hypoxemia — Inadequate oxygen supply in the arterial blood.

Hypoxia — Inadequate oxygen supply to the body tissues.

Larynx — The organ of voice production; also known as the voice box.

Mediastinum — The space within the chest, located between the lungs, that contains the heart, major blood vessels, trachea and esophagus.

Patent Foramen Ovale *(PFO)* — A hole in the septum *(wall)* between the right and left atria *(upper chambers)* of the heart.

Pericardium — A double-layered membranous sac surrounding the heart and the major blood vessels connected to it.

Pharynx — Portion of the airway connecting nasal cavity and larynx.

Pleura — Membrane surrounding the outer surface of the lungs, the inner surface of the chest wall and the diaphragm.

Surfactant — A substance produced in the lungs to reduce surface tension in alveoli and small airways.

Thorax — The upper part of the trunk between the neck and the abdomen which contains the heart, lungs, trachea and bronchi.

Trachea — The air passage that begins at the larynx and ends as the beginning of the principal right and left bronchi.

Ventricle — Thick-walled, muscular chamber which receives blood from the atrium, pumping it through to pulmonary or systemic circulation.

Venules — Small veins.

Oxygen First Aid Anatomy & Physiology

Oxygen is beneficial for the successful outcome for diving injuries.

Oxygen first aid provided to the injured diver prior to the arrival of professional medical care is one of the most important measures taken when a diving injury occurs.

In the special situation of the diving injury, there is an important role for oxygen. The most common diving injuries are arterial gas embolism (AGE) and decompression sickness *(DCS)*. These injuries are caused by bubbles — AGE by bubbles that enter the arterial circulation through the lungs, and DCS by bubbles that form in the body tissues.

Bubbles in blood vessels result in blockage or reduction of oxygenated blood supply. If blood supply to the brain is interrupted, permanent damage or death may occur. The prompt use of 100 percent inhaled oxygen may reduce bubble size by removing nitrogen from the body tissues and blood and will help supply oxygen to areas of the body where this supply has been reduced.

A pressure gradient from the nitrogen bubble to the tissues is created so the bubble may become smaller or even disappear, allowing circulation to improve. Effective elimination of nitrogen and reduction of bubble size will restore oxygenated blood flow to hypoxic tissues.

There are many conditions that may prevent adequate oxygen supply to the tissues. There may be medical illnesses such as chronic lung or heart disease causing the problem. A past injury may interfere with respiration. Obstruction of the upper airway by a foreign body or the tongue in the unresponsive injured diver is common. Lung expansion injuries frequently cause shortness of breath and difficulty breathing and require oxygen to improve oxygen supply to the body tissues. The injured diver who has experienced a near-drowning may have water in the lungs and require high oxygen concentrations.

The DAN Oxygen Provider course emphasizes the use of oxygen for diving injuries, but does not address many other indications for oxygen treatment.

Respiration and Circulation

It is important to understand the anatomy and function of the circulatory and respiratory systems in order to recognize the role of oxygen. The physical process of breathing is so constant that its existence is rarely noticed. However, if breathing is interrupted for even a few minutes and not restored, stages of severe discomfort, unconsciousness, irreversible brain damage and, eventually death, occur.

By understanding the structures of the respiratory system and the process of breathing, you will be able to select a proper course of first aid for a diver requiring supplemental oxygen. You will also be able to apply this knowledge to your use of oxygen in an emergency situation.

The respiratory system primarily deals with the exchange of oxygen and carbon dioxide between the bloodstream and the environment. However, the exchange of inert gases such as nitrogen, which plays no significant role in metabolism and waste gases such as carbon dioxide, also occurs through the respiratory system. As long as air is breathed, you will always have an amount of nitrogen dissolved in your body that is directly proportional to the partial pressure of nitrogen in the air.

Other gases such as carbon monoxide *(CO)* can interfere with the process of breathing. Carbon monoxide is present in minute quantities throughout the atmosphere. Carbon monoxide binds to the hemoglobin preventing oxygen from being absorbed by the blood.

The body requires a constant supply of oxygen for the body cells to run the metabolic machinery. In the absence of oxygen *(a condition known as anoxia)*, the body's cells will deteriorate and die. Some cells are more sensitive than others to the deficiency of oxygen depending on their function and location — the cells of the brain and nervous system, for example, are very sensitive and will die within a few minutes of being deprived of oxygen.

Carbon dioxide is produced in the cells during the metabolism of oxygen and returns to the lungs in the bloodstream as a waste product. Most of the carbon dioxide produced by the body is eliminated through exhalation, but there is a normal level of carbon dioxide in the blood. Respiratory centers in the brain

By understanding the structures of the respiratory system and the process of breathing, you will be able to select a proper course of first aid for a diver requiring supplemental oxygen.

Airway and Respiratory System

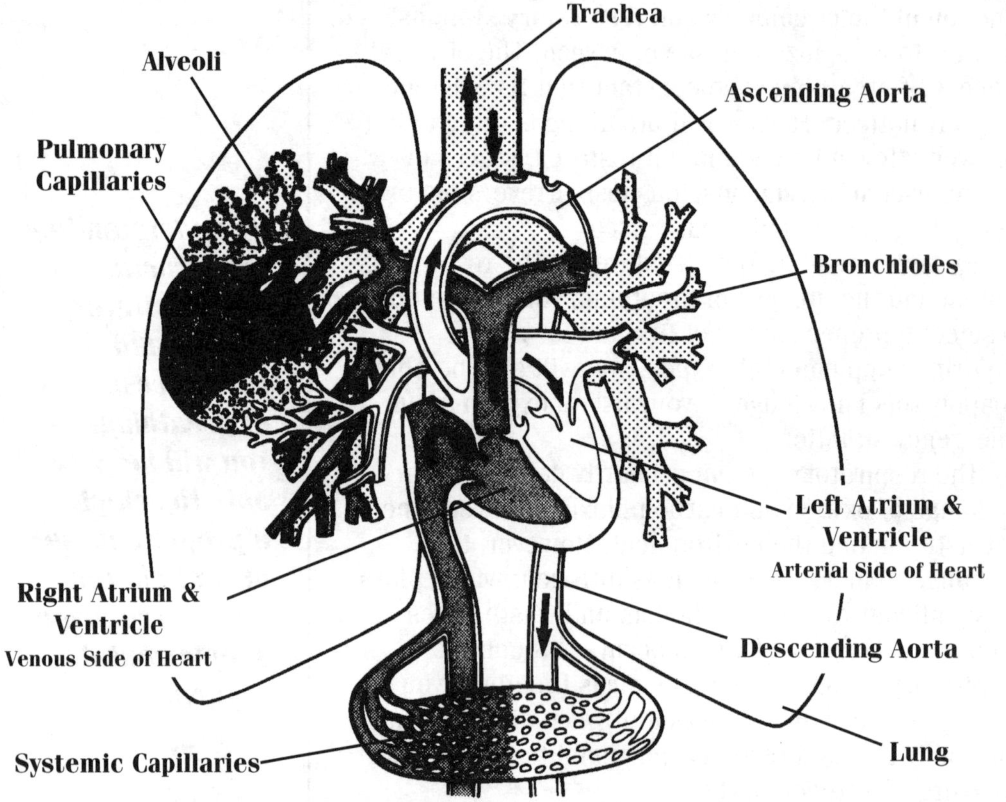

Respiratory centers in the brain respond to the level of carbon dioxide in the bloodstream which initiates and regulates the rate and depth of respiration.

respond to the level of carbon dioxide in the bloodstream which initiates and regulates the rate and depth of respiration. If the level of carbon dioxide goes up, the rate and depth of respirations will increase, and if the level goes down, the opposite will happen. There are centers in the circulatory system that respond to a lack of oxygen in the blood supply. However, their signal is usually ineffective during respiratory arrest, and hypoxia *(inadequate supply of oxygen to body tissues)* will result unless normal breathing is restored.

This system is extremely important for diving. If the oxygen level is too low in the breathing mixture *(a rare circumstance in recreational diving)*, unconsciousness and death due to hypoxia may occur without the diver being aware of the problem.

The functions of the respiratory and circulatory systems are so closely related that they must be considered together. The respiratory system provides a mechanism to bring blood and gases that make up the breathing medium together *(without actually physically mixing)* so that gas exchange can occur.

Gas exchange is the uptake of oxygen from the lungs and removal of carbon dioxide from the blood. The circulatory system then transports oxygen to all the tissues of the body where another series of gas exchanges occur. This time oxygen passes from the blood to the tissues, and carbon dioxide returns from the working tissues to the blood.

Gas exchange is the uptake of oxygen from the lungs and removal of carbon dioxide from the blood.

The Respiratory System

The respiratory system consists of the ribs, intercostal *(between the ribs)* muscles, diaphragm, lungs, mouth and nose and a series of pipes connecting the mouth and nose with the lungs. The lungs, situated in the chest cavity *(or thorax)*, are roughly cone-shaped. They are composed of elastic tissue; each is surrounded by two very thin membranes called the pleura. One membrane covers the lung itself and the other, the chest wall. The space enclosed between the pleura is called the pleural cavity. This area contains a thin layer of fluid that acts as a lubricant to allow efficient movement of the lungs during breathing.

Air is drawn into the mouth and nose and passes into the pharynx, which is a short common passageway for air and food. The pharynx divides into two tubes — the trachea *(windpipe)* and the esophagus.

The esophagus is located behind the trachea and takes food and fluids into the stomach. Air travels through the larynx *(voice box)* and into the trachea. The epiglottis, a flexible flap of tissue and cartilage located at the back of the tongue, prevents food from entering the larynx by folding over the larynx during swallowing.

The trachea is composed of a series of semicircular cartilaginous rings that prevent collapse. It passes down into the chest cavity and divides into two tubes, the right and left bronchi, which enter the right and left lungs, respectively. Inside the lungs, the bronchi progressively divide into smaller and smaller tubes like the branches of a tree. The smaller branches of the respiratory tree also are supported by cartilage.

Alveoli are located at the end of the smallest branches of the respiratory tree. They have extremely thin walls and are surrounded in basket-like fashion by the pulmonary capillaries. The alveoli have been likened to tiny balloons or clusters of grapes.

In both lungs, there are millions of alveoli with a combined surface area of more than 1,000 square feet /93 square meters — or roughly the size of a tennis court.

Actual physical damage to the lungs may not be necessary for gases to pass through the alveoli into the bloodstream.

The inner surfaces of the alveoli are coated with a detergent-like substance known as a surfactant. This surfactant acts to decrease the surface tension of the alveoli, thereby reducing their tendency to collapse. If the surfactant were to dissolve, as may occur in near-drowning, the alveoli may collapse.

The air-filled alveoli are only one micrometer (0.000039 inch) in diameter *(roughly 1/20th of the thickness of this page)*. The barrier between gas and blood, only one cell thick, is called the alveolar-capillary membrane. If the alveolar-capillary membrane is torn or damaged, a lung overpressure injury may result. Actual physical damage may not be necessary for gases to pass through the alveoli into the bloodstream. Movement of gas across the alveolar membrane into the capillary system may occur without causing any perceptible tissue damage.

The blood's primary purpose is to carry gases and nutrients.

The trachea and bronchi are lined with cells that have tiny hairlike bodies *(known as cilia)* on their surface. These cilia, along with mucus secreted by glands, act to trap foreign particles and move them up into the pharynx where they are subsequently swallowed. Cilia are damaged or deactivated by exposure to nicotine. Chronic smokers must resort to the "smoker's cough" to rid their lungs of mucous buildup and foreign particles. Mucous buildup may predispose a diver to gas-trapping.

The Cardiovascular System

The cardiovascular system consists of the heart and blood vessels. This system is a closed-circuit system designed to transport a fluid called blood. The blood's primary purpose is to carry gases and nutrients.

The Heart

The heart is a hollow muscular organ situated in the chest between the lungs in a space called the mediastinum. The heart, like the lungs, is surrounded by a thin connective tissue sac, the pericardium, that allows the heart to beat independently without friction. The heart is situated obliquely, one-third to the right and two-thirds to the left of the sternum.

The heart is a strong muscular pump that, in the average adult, beats about 70 times per minute. Every minute, approximately 6 liters *(6.34 quarts)* of blood is pumped throughout the body. When exercising, this output doubles or triples depending upon the amount of exertion.

The heart consists of two separate pumps, one on the left side of the heart and one on the right side. Each pump has two chambers. The upper chamber, or atrium, receives blood from the body or the lungs, and the lower chamber, the ventricle, is filled with blood from the atrium. The pumps work by muscular contraction squeezing the blood out of the chambers. The left ventricle pumps oxygenated blood throughout the body in what is known as the systemic circuit, and the right ventricle pumps deoxygenated blood to the lungs in what is known as the pulmonary circuit.

The left ventricle pumps oxygenated blood throughout the body in what is known as the systemic circuit, and the right ventricle pumps deoxygenated blood to the lungs in what is known as the pulmonary circuit.

In the fetus, the lungs are not fully functional. The blood bypasses the lungs, the majority passing directly from the right atrium to the left atrium through a natural opening called the foramen ovale. At birth, when the pressure in the left atrium becomes slightly greater than the right, a "flap" valve closes over the foramen ovale *(the remnant structure known as the fossa ovalis)* allowing the blood to be pumped directly to the lungs. In some individuals, the closure is incomplete and the result is a patent *(or open)* foramen ovale *(PFO)*.

This condition may allow blood to flow from the left to the right atrium or vice versa. Divers with a PFO are generally unaware of it, and under normal circumstances, it may cause no problems at all.

Some data suggest, however, that in some divers, bubbles may be allowed to pass directly from the right to the left atrium and into the arterial circulation. The result is that bubbles may enter the cerebral circulation with resultant cerebral or cardiac *(similar to a heart attack)* manifestations of DCI. In addition, if the diver performs the Valsalva maneuver when diving *(the forced inflation of the middle ear by exhaling with the mouth closed and the nostrils pinched)*, right-to-left shunting may be precipitated, or enhanced, during the release phase of the maneuver.

The blood carries oxygen in two forms: one is dissolved in plasma, the other chemically combined with hemoglobin.

Blood Vessels

When blood leaves the left ventricle, it passes into the aorta, which is the largest artery of the body. It has thick elastic walls that recoil during ventricular relaxation to maintain arterial pressure while the ventricle refills. The aorta branches to all parts of the body. Blood leaving the right ventricle passes into the pulmonary trunk, which divides almost immediately into the right and left pulmonary arteries. These transport deoxygenated blood to the lungs for gas exchange.

The blood vessels make up the vascular tree, with each branch giving rise to progressively smaller branches. The smallest arteries are called arterioles, and it is from these that the capillaries, the smallest of all blood vessels, arise.

The arterioles have the job of controlling blood flow to the capillaries. The capillaries are the business end of the entire cardiovascular system. It is through these thin walls that gases and nutrients are exchanged — the heart and large blood vessels are only a pump and distribution system for the capillaries.

From the capillaries, the blood is gathered into small, thin-walled veins *(called venules)* and returned via larger veins to the atria of the heart. Most veins direct blood flow by means of one-way valves that prevent blood from traveling in the wrong direction.

Gas Exchange

Oxygen constitutes approximately 21 percent of air. Oxygen is required to metabolize food and to provide energy for cell function. The body consumes oxygen and produces heat and other forms of energy and carbon dioxide.

Exhaled air contains approximately 16 percent oxygen. The blood carries oxygen in two forms: one is dissolved in plasma, the other chemically combined with hemoglobin *(called oxyhemoglobin)*. Due to the high binding capacity of hemoglobin, oxygen is not very soluble in plasma at normal temperatures and surface pressures; therefore, the vast majority of oxygen is bound to hemoglobin.

The inert gas nitrogen, which has no part in metabolism, consists of about 78 percent of air. Since the body does not use nitrogen, exhaled air also contains about 78 percent nitrogen.

When breathing air at normal atmospheric pressure, the hemoglobin is 97.5 percent saturated with oxygen. As the oxygen-rich blood reaches the tissues, the hemoglobin releases some oxygen but still remains about 75 percent saturated. The oxygen is released from the hemoglobin because the partial pressure of oxygen in the tissues is lower than in the blood. According to diffusion laws, gas moves from areas of high partial pressure to areas of low partial pressure.

Gas moves from areas of high partial pressure to areas of low partial pressure.

Inhaled air contains about 0.033 percent carbon dioxide. Carbon dioxide is a waste product of our metabolism and is carried in our blood in three ways. A small amount *(approximately 8 percent)* is dissolved in the plasma, another small amount *(11 percent)* is bound to hemoglobin or plasma proteins, but most of the carbon dioxide *(81 percent)* in our blood is carried as bicarbonate. Exhaled gas from respiration contains approximately 4 percent carbon dioxide.

Blood

Blood can be considered an intermediary in the functioning of the respiratory and circulatory systems. The body contains 4 to 6 liters *(4.23 to 6.34 quarts)* of blood, the actual amount depending upon body size and gender, with females having a lower blood volume than males.

Blood cells are formed in the bone marrow. Red blood cells *(RBCs)*, also called erythrocytes, live for approximately 120 days and are then removed by the spleen. White blood cells *(WBCs)*, called leukocytes, live from six hours to a year, depending on the type of cell and its function. Red blood cell formation is controlled by a hormone that is produced by the kidneys. Reduced oxygen levels, that can be caused, for example, by living at altitude, increase the production of red blood cells.

Review Questions

1. Hypoxia results when there is an insufficient supply of oxygen delivered to body tissues.

a. True   b. False

2. Air contains approximately _____ % oxygen and _____ % nitrogen. Exhaled air contains _____ % oxygen.

a. 21, 78, 16   b. 16, 78, 21
c. 20, 80, 20   d. 16, 78, 21

3. Gas exchange takes place in the ________.

a. arterioles   b. aorta
c. alveoli   d. atrium

4. The respiratory system consists of the ribs, diaphragm, lungs, mouth, nose and heart.

a. True   b. False

5. The circulatory system consists of the heart and blood vessels and is designed to carry gases and nutrients via blood.

a. True   b. False

Answers
1.a
2.a
3.c
4.b
5.a

Diving Injuries

KEY TERMS

Arterial Gas Embolism *(AGE)* — Gas bubbles in the arterial system generally caused by air passing through the walls of the alveoli in the lungs into the bloodstream.

Barotrauma — Injury that results from changes in surrounding pressure.

Central Nervous System *(CNS)* — Division of the nervous system containing the brain and spinal cord.

Cyanosis — Bluish or purplish discoloration of the skin due to insufficient oxygenation of the blood.

Decompression Illness *(DCI)* — Dysbaric injuries related to scuba diving; includes both arterial gas embolism and decompression sickness.

Decompression Sickness *(DCS)* — A syndrome caused by bubbles of inert gas forming in the tissues and bloodstream which can evolve from a rapid ascent from compressed gas diving, or a reduction in surrounding pressure such as flying in an aircraft.

Drowning — Suffocation in water or other liquid.

Edema — An abnormal excess accumulation of fluid; swelling.

Extremity — A limb of the body.

Hyperbaric Oxygen Therapy — Treatment where patient breathes 100 percent oxygen intermittently while pressure is increased to a point higher than sea level.

Mean — Average.

Median — A value in an ordered set of values below and above which there is an equal number of values.

Near-drowning — Survival after suffocation in water or other liquid.

Occlude — To close off or stop up; obstruct.

Sign — Any medical or trauma condition that can be observed and described.

Symptom — Any non-observable condition described by the patient.

OBJECTIVES

In this chapter you'll learn to

1. **Describe the difference between a sign and a symptom.**
2. **State the three most common diving injuries.**
3. **List at least five common diving injury signs and symptoms.**
4. **Describe at least five common diving injury signs and symptoms.**
5. **State the common onset times for DCI.**

The Mechanism of Diving Injuries

Drowning

Drowning occurs when water is inhaled into the lungs, impairing the body's ability to transfer oxygen into the bloodstream. Drowning leads to hypoxia. The presence of water in the lungs damages the alveoli and causes them to collapse. The collapsed alveoli are no longer able to exchange oxygen and carbon dioxide in the blood. An insult *(injury)* to the lungs, whether it is the introduction of water or for other reasons, may result in pulmonary edema (the release of fluid into the lungs). Near-drowning results in a vast array of signs and symptoms, including unconsciousness, chest pain, dizziness, cyanosis *(bluish coloration)*, shortness of breath, coughing, frothy sputum and death. The injured diver experiencing near-drowning symptoms requires high concentrations of inhaled oxygen to minimize the damaging effects of hypoxia.

What about other pulmonary barotrauma?

Signs and symptoms for pulmonary barotrauma other than AGE include:

- difficulty breathing,
- chest pain,
- cyanosis,
- swelling of the neck area,
- voice changes, and
- crackling under the skin.

Since AGE is the most serious of the lung overexpansion injuries and may accompany other pulmonary barotrauma, it is important to try **not** to differentiate between them and provide appropriate care.

Decompression Illness *(DCI)*

The mechanism of decompression illness is bubble formation and growth, resulting in oxygen deficiency, or hypoxia. Decompression illness encompasses two conditions: decompression sickness *(DCS)*, commonly referred to as the bends; and arterial gas embolism (AGE), commonly referred to as air embolism. Because the symptoms of both injuries are similar and because both conditions require the same first aid and treatment, this term is being used more frequently in the diving community.

Because the first aid and initial treatment for both DCS and AGE are identical, avoid trying to differentiate between the two injuries. It is more important that the symptoms are recognized when they occur after a dive. Remember, a diving injury can occur following a dive to any depth, and there may be no apparent reason for the injury.

Arterial Gas Embolism *(AGE)*

Arterial gas embolism may occur as a result of a lung overpressure injury while breathing compressed air and ascending from a dive. Air, which is introduced into the bloodstream in the lungs, returns to the heart, blocking major arteries or may pass directly to the

Arterial Gas Embolism

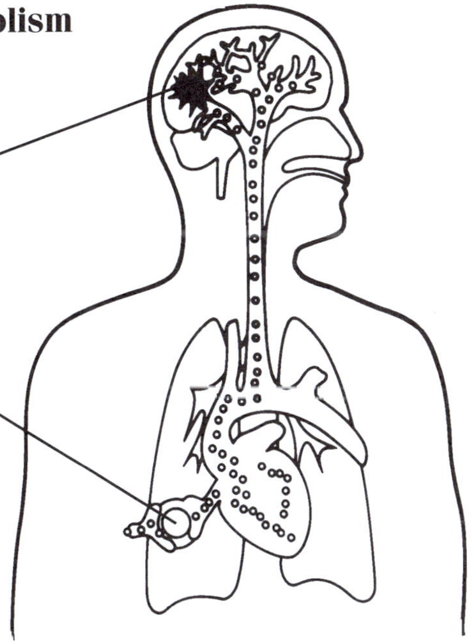

brain, causing rapid and dramatic symptoms. Although AGE can occur for no apparent reason, common contributing factors may include rapid ascent, breath-holding, lung congestion, asthma, lung damage or other air-trapping conditions. Signs and symptoms for pulmonary barotrauma other than AGE include difficulty breathing, chest pain, cyanosis, swelling of the neck area, voice changes and crackling under the skin.

Since AGE is the most serious of the lung over-expansion injuries and may accompany other pulmonary barotrauma, it is important to try not to differentiate between them and provide appropriate care.

Decompression Sickness *(DCS)*

Decompression sickness is a result of bubbles that form and grow during or after ascent as a result of excess nitrogen *(or other inert gas)* absorbed by the tissues during diving activities. Bubbles can have mechanical or biochemical effects. Mechanical effects include distortion or tearing of tissue and reduction or stoppage of blood flow. Biochemical effects include activation of clotting and inflammatory mechanisms, with resulting leakage of fluids out of the circulatory system and narrowing of vessels.

Bubbles cause different problems depending on their location: pain, if in the joints; sensory or motor dysfunction, if in the spinal cord; shortness of breath or breathing difficulty, if in the lungs; and impairment of hearing, speech, thought or consciousness, if in the brain. Perhaps the most dangerous form of DCS is triggered by an air embolism at the end of a dive. Arterial bubbles entering the brain or spinal cord expand rapidly from the excess absorbed nitrogen. This diver can have it all: cerebral, spinal and joint DCS.

Life-threatening signs do occur but are not common. Sometimes signs and symptoms will go away without treatment, but early treatment is strongly advised as the chance of permanent injury becomes greater with delayed or omitted treatment. Providing 100 percent inhaled oxygen as soon as signs or symptoms are noted and during transportation to definitive medical care is essential and improves the probability of complete recovery.

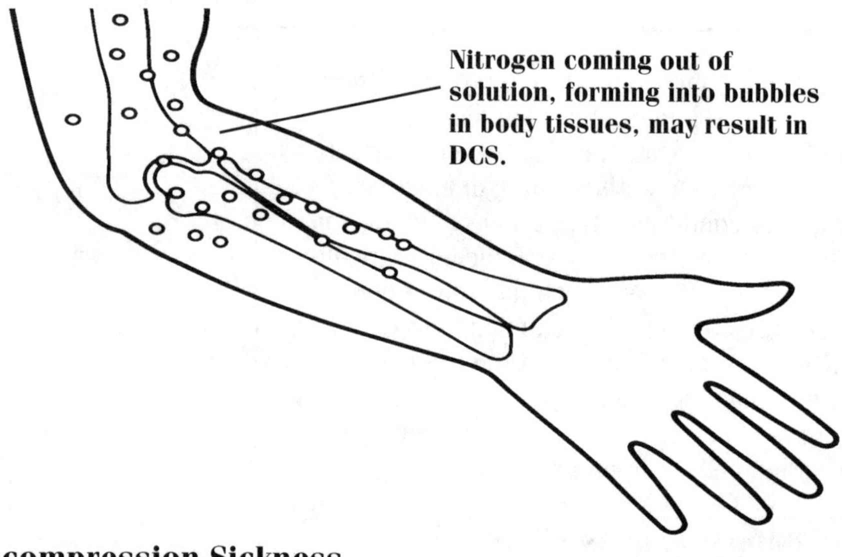

Decompression Sickness

Signs and Symptoms

The recognition of decompression illness is based on an individual's recent history of scuba diving and the presence of signs and symptoms. DCI has a broad range of symptoms that can mimic many known illnesses and injuries.

A symptom is a subjective complaint of which only the injured diver is aware such as discomfort, aches and pains and general ill feeling. A sign is an objective finding that can be seen or demonstrated on physical examination such as weakness or limping. Although any sign or symptom may signal DCI, it's important to listen for comments the injured diver may make about potential symptoms and watch for signs as a DAN Oxygen Provider.

Nature of DCI

Decompression illness has no definitive presentation or test to confirm its presence. There is often no outward sign of injury that would indicate either mild or severe symptoms. Any area of the body may be involved.

Symptoms may be very vague and subtle and are often initially dismissed by the diver. Symptoms can resolve spontaneously before a diver reports them or reaches medical care.

If 100 percent oxygen is used as emergency first aid, the symptoms may also resolve. However, symptom resolution does not rule out the need for physical evaluation by a trained healthcare professional and possible treatment at a hyperbaric facility. Additional symptoms can go undetected or become worse. Also, symptoms can return after initial resolution, either with or without treatment. Fatigue, anxiety, emotional stress, or physical exertion may facilitate their return. For this reason, divers are always advised to seek medical evaluation if they suspect they are injured.

A sign is an objective finding that can be seen or demonstrated on physical examination, such as weakness or limping.

A symptom is a subjective complaint of which only the diver is aware, such as discomfort, aches and pains, and a general ill feeling.

Common Signs and Symptoms

Injured divers may have just one of the following signs and symptoms, or they may have several at the same time. DCI is unpredictable.

Common Signs & Symptoms of DCI

- **Numbness**
- **Headache**
- **Dizziness**
- **Nausea**
- **Pain**
- **Weakness**
- **Unusual Fatigue**
- **Difficulty Walking**

Other Signs & Symptoms of DCI

- ✦ **Difficutly Breathing**
- ✦ **Visual Disturbance**
- ✦ **Decreased Skin Sensation**
- ✦ **Restlessness**
- ✦ **Itching/Rash**
- ✦ **Paralysis**
- ✦ **Muscle Twitching**
- ✦ **Unconsciousness**
- ✦ **Speech Disturbance**
- ✦ **Personality Change**
- ✦ **Altered Level of Consciousness**
- ✦ **Bladder/Bowel Problems**
- ✦ **Convulsions**
- ✦ **Hearing Loss/Ringing Ears**
- ✦ **Coughing Blood**

Descriptions of Common Signs and Symptoms

It is important for DAN Oxygen Providers to understand the more common and the most serious signs and symptoms of DCI and their descriptions.

• *Pain*

Pain can be a dull, sharp, boring or aching sensation in or around a joint or muscle. A pain may be so mild that it is no more than a sensation. It may begin gradually and build in intensity. Movement of the effected joint or limb may or may not make a difference in the severity of the pain. The pain may be out of proportion to the amount of work or exercise the diver associates with the discomfort and may be referred to as unusual or just a "different" type of pain. DCI pain can be difficult to distinguish from the "miseries of daily life." Symptoms can mimic other illness such as viral infections, muscle or joint pain, fatigue from exertion, and other nonspecific discomforts.

• *Numbness and Tingling*

This sensation is sometimes referred to as "pins and needles." A diver may complain of feeling as though an extremity has fallen "asleep" or a "funny bone" has been hit. Numbness and tingling most often occurs in the limbs and may be associated with complaints such as cold, heavy or swollen sensations. Numbness and tingling may start in the hands or feet and gradually move up the extremity.

• *Dizziness*

Dizziness or vertigo generally refers to a sense of spinning. It can lead to a loss of balance requiring a diver to walk with assistance or the diver may even fall. Like headaches, dizziness may be associated with other CNS signs or symptoms and is serious. Dizziness can be caused by DCI or ear barotrauma. Both require early medical evaluation and treatment to increase the chance of full recovery. Evaluation is particularly important, as treatment for the two conditions is different.

• *Extreme Fatigue*

It is not unusual to be fatigued after a scuba dive or other physical exertion. The fatigue associated with DCI is more severe and out of proportion with the exercise of the dive. The diver may describe this as a fatigue they have never felt before. The diver may want to lie down or sleep and may ignore personal responsibilities such as stowing gear or cleaning equipment. Friends may describe the diver's behavior as unusual.

• *Headache*

Post-dive headaches are common and ambiguous. While they may be due to too much sun, they also can represent sinus barotrauma or central nervous system *(CNS)* decompression illness. Headaches from DCI are often accompanied by other symptoms that may affect the higher functions like speech, hearing, personality and thinking.

• *Nausea*

Nausea is the overwhelming sensation prior to vomiting. There may be causes other than DCI for nausea, such as seasickness.

• *Difficulty Walking*

Difficulty walking can be caused by dizziness, nausea, weakness of a limb, generalized weakness, paralysis or impaired mental status. A diver may lean on others to maintain balance or move from object to object in order to support himself or herself. An altered gait such as a limp or the sliding of one foot may also indicate walking difficulty. In the worst case, total lower extremity paralysis may be present.

> ***DAN Membership and Dive Accident Insurance provides:***
>
> **DAN *TravelAssist,*** which provides access to potential evacuation in a medical emergency when traveling; and
>
> **DAN insurance,** which offers affordable and comprehensive dive accident insurance in the unlikely event of diving injury. Various choices are available.
>
> Ask your DAN Oxygen Instructor for more information, or contact the DAN office in your region.

• *Altered Skin Sensation*

Altered skin sensation may represent either decreased or lost sensation or hypersensitivity (increased sensitivity) where light touch causes discomfort. Loss of sensation may only effect a small patch of skin such as the back of the shoulder or side of the thigh and may not be noticed unless the diver bumps or injures the affected area. Decreased sensation is indicated by difficulty in detecting a difference between objects that are sharp and dull or soft and hard.

• *Rash and Itching*

Rash and itching may occur together but may not be caused by DCI. Itching due to DCI may last for minutes to hours and may affect an entire limb or just small area of the body. A rash due to DCI may be localized or spread over a wide area such as the chest or shoulder and may be pink or red. It may also have a marbled appearance much like a bruise and occur over areas such as the abdomen, thighs, chest, upper arms and shoulders.

Trends in Dive Accidents

Few of the dive accidents reported to DAN are of a catastrophic nature. Diving injuries that result in a non-breathing diver are rare. However, it should be noted that there is an average of 95 recreational scuba diving fatalities a year reported to DAN America, including U.S. and Canadian citizens.

Symptom Onset Time

Decompression illness usually involves multiple symptoms that occur at different times. The onset of signs and symptoms of DCI vary from during the dive to 24 hours or more after the dive.

The median symptom onset time for AGE is one minute for both the first and second symptom. This means that in some cases, the injured diver may experience symptoms while still on the surface or possibly under the water, which could lead to drowning.

The signs and symptoms of DCS evolve more slowly than those of AGE. The median symptom onset time is one hour after surfacing. However, since symptoms have been reported to appear greater than

24 hours after the dive, you need to be alert for anything suspicious, even hours after a dive.

It is important to note that many divers with decompression illness continue to dive after developing the first signs and symptoms. The reasons for this are not well documented. However, it may be due to a lack of symptom recognition or a reluctance to mention symptoms in a group of peers.

Evidence suggests that post-dive activities such as physical exertion and altitude exposure may contribute to the development of DCI symptoms.

DAN suggests that divers carry dive accident insurance in order to be prepared for a diving injury. The costs of evacuation and medical treatments for diving injuries can be quite high and are often not covered in personal healthcare plans.

Delay to Call and Recompression Treatment

Frequently there is a considerable delay from symptom onset time to calling for assistance and subsequent treatment. There are many reasons divers delay seeking medical evaluation or assistance. Signs and symptoms of decompression illness can be very subtle and may go unnoticed for a considerable period of time. Some individuals may prefer not to seek evaluation due to the remote locations, or they do not feel their symptoms are serious enough to seek treatment. Often divers claim to be concerned about the expense of evacuation and treatment which may contribute to unnecessary delay.

An injured diver may feel better or have symptoms improve after receiving oxygen first aid, but because of the high incidence of recurrence of symptoms following oxygen first aid, evaluation by a qualified physician and possible hyperbaric treatment may still be required. The longer a diver delays evaluation and treatment for a dive accident, the lower the chances are of effective treatment and complete symptom resolution.

Residual Symptoms After Treatment

Post-treatment residual symptoms are frequently described by injured divers. The reasons for this are unclear and are still being studied.

It is important that a diver who is experiencing residual symptoms following hyperbaric oxygen treatment should not resume diving until all symptoms have resolved. In addition, the diver should be cleared to dive by a physician knowledgeable in diving medicine before resuming diving activities.

Review Questions

1. An injured diver is seen holding and rubbing his/her shoulder following a dive. This is a _______.

a. Sign b. Symptom

2. A diver complains of a headache following a dive. This is a _______.

a. Sign b. Symptom

3. Any sign or symptom following a dive may signal decompression illness.

a. True b. False

4. List five common signs or symptoms of decompression illness.

a. _______________
b. _______________
c. _______________
d. _______________
e. _______________

5. Most signs and symptoms present during the first two hours following a dive.

a. True b. False

Answers

1. a
2. b
3. a
4. Numbness, Pain, Dizziness, Unusual Fatigue, Headache, Weakness, Nausea, Difficulty Walking, Difficulty Breathing, Itching, Rash, Paralysis, Bladder or Bowel Problems, Decreased Skin Sensation, Unconsciousness, Hearing Loss/Ringing Ears
5. a

Oxygen and Its Hazards

KEY TERMS

Central Nervous System *(CNS)* — The division of the nervous system containing the brain and spinal cord.

Fractional distillation — Vaporizing by heat and condensing and collecting into portions, parts or fractions.

Prescription — A written order for dispensing drugs signed by a physician.

Pulmonary — Concerning or involving the lungs.

OBJECTIVES

In this chapter you'll learn to

1. **Name the minimum grade of oxygen suitable for breathing.**
2. **List two potential hazards of breathing high concentrations of oxygen.**
3. **List at least two risks associated with the handling of oxygen cylinders.**
4. **List two common requirements for obtaining an oxygen cylinder fill.**

Oxygen

The key supporting element of life is oxygen. The cells of the body require a constant supply of oxygen. It is a colorless, odorless and tasteless gas and comprises approximately 21 percent of the atmosphere. Oxygen alone is capable of supporting life and can be used for short periods of time as a breathing medium instead of air. High concentrations of oxygen are commonly used for medical purposes.

In normal respiration, approximately 21 percent oxygen is required at one atmosphere to carry out normal daily living needs. If the percentage of oxygen decreases in the breathing air, body function can be affected. Brain cells, nerve cells and heart muscle are most susceptible to the lack of oxygen, which is referred to as hypoxia. In response to hypoxia, the body will increase the heart rate and raise the blood pressure in an effort to bring more oxygen from the lungs. The use of emergency oxygen assists in getting oxygen to the body's hypoxic tissues.

Where Does Pure Oxygen Come From?

Pure oxygen is obtained by fractional distillation of air. Air is first filtered to remove any debris and dirt. It is then compressed to very high pressures and dried to remove water vapor. To liquefy the gas, it is cooled to very low temperatures and then allowed to slowly rewarm. As it is rewarming, the various components of air *(oxygen and nitrogen primarily)* are captured and stored in separate containers as they reach their particular boiling points.

Use only medical- or higher-grade oxygen for diving injuries. Industrial-grade oxygen is not recommended for breathing.

There are many grades of oxygen, but the three primary ones that DAN Oxygen Providers need to consider are:

- aviator-grade,
- medical-grade, and
- industrial-grade oxygen.

These three oxygen grades are required to be 99.5 percent pure oxygen. However, there are differences in how the cylinders are filled. The differences affect the overall purity of the oxygen. For example, aviator-grade oxygen has a lower moisture content than the medical grade, to prevent freezing at high altitudes.

The filling procedures for medical-grade oxygen require that an odor test is conducted and the cylinder contents evacuated prior to filling. When odors are detected or damage to the valve or cylinder is observed, medical-grade oxygen cylinders are cleaned prior to returning them to use.

Industrial-grade oxygen is not recommended for use for diving injuries. Industrial-grade oxygen guidelines allow for a certain percentage of impurities and other gases to be contained within the cylinder. While both aviator- and medical-grade oxygen are suitable for breathing, industrial-grade may not be. The procedures for filling of industrial oxygen cylinders do not ensure that the oxygen is free of contamination.

Hazards of Breathing Oxygen

Oxygen poisoning, or toxicity, can occur by breathing high oxygen concentrations. There are two forms of oxygen toxicity: central nervous system *(CNS)* and pulmonary *(lung)* toxicity. In CNS oxygen toxicity, seizures may develop when oxygen is breathed at greater than one atmosphere absolute pressure. Breathing high concentrations of oxygen at the surface can cause pulmonary oxygen toxicity. Damage occurs to the alveoli in the lungs from breathing 100 percent oxygen over a period of days. Pulmonary oxygen toxicity usually takes longer in individuals with healthy lung tissue. Oxygen toxicity is generally not a concern for the Oxygen Provider rendering first aid. However, if the injured diver is five hours or more away from the nearest appropriate medical center, it may be important to allow for short interruptions for the breathing of air when breathing high concentrations of oxygen to reduce the risks of oxygen toxicity.

Hazards of Handling Oxygen

Oxygen is not flammable, but all substances need oxygen to burn — and may burn violently in an environment of pure oxygen. Problems associated with the use of properly maintained emergency oxygen devices are rare. Three elements are required for a fire to exist and they are heat, fuel and oxygen. This is commonly called the fire triangle. Emergency oxygen systems will always have at least one element and that is oxygen. As a DAN Oxygen Provider, you need to reduce the risks of handling oxygen. Be sure that the hazards from both the fuel, *(oil deposits and hydrocarbons, commonly used as lubricants for diving and found on dive boats)* and heat from sun and rapid opening of the oxygen cylinder valve are minimized.

As a DAN Oxygen Provider, you need to reduce the risks of handling oxygen.

Safety Precautions When Using Oxygen

Oxygen cylinders require the same care as scuba cylinders, with a few additional precautions.

- ✦ *Do not allow the use of any oil or grease on any cylinder or device that comes in contact with oxygen. The result may be a fire.*
- ✦ *Oxygen cylinders should not be exposed to temperatures over 125° F or 52° C in storage (for example, a car trunk).*
- ✦ *Do not allow smoking or an open flame around oxygen and oxygen equipment.*
- ✦ *Remember to provide adequate ventilation when using oxygen. In a confined, poorly ventilated space (like in the cabin of a boat), the oxygen concentration may build up and create a fire hazard.*
- ✦ *Only equipment (cylinders, regulators, valves and gauges) intended for use with oxygen should be used. Avoid adapting scuba equipment for use with oxygen.*
- ✦ *Visually inspect the condition of valve seats and oxygen washers and make sure the materials are compatible for oxygen use.*
- ✦ *Valves should remain closed with the system purged when the unit is not in use. Valves on empty cylinders should be closed. Empty cylinders should be refilled immediately after use.*

- *An oxygen cylinder should always be secured so that it cannot fall. When carrying an oxygen cylinder by hand, carry it with both hands and avoid holding it by the valve or regulator. When transporting an oxygen cylinder in a car, secure and block the cylinder so it does not roll.*

- *Oxygen cylinders require hydrostatic testing periodically just as scuba cylinders do. Be sure the test date is within the required time.*

To be filled, oxygen cylinders generally require either: 1) a prescription, or 2) documentation of training.

Oxygen Cylinder Filling

In many areas, medical grade oxygen is considered a drug. As a drug, it may be difficult to obtain oxygen for your emergency oxygen cylinder. The most common method of documenting the need for oxygen is a prescription. However, prescriptions are for diagnosed medical conditions. The prescription allows for use only by the individual who was given the prescription.

The other method of obtaining an oxygen cylinder fill is by providing documentation of training in the use of emergency oxygen. Like your scuba diving certification card, your DAN Oxygen Provider card is your documentation of appropriate training. Since retraining is recommended every two years, you will need to maintain your skills by taking an oxygen refresher program. Ask your Oxygen Instructor about retraining opportunities.

Some countries, states and local governments have regulations that require that oxygen supply companies document all medical grade oxygen distillation, cylinder transfills and sales. These governmental agencies routinely inspect the facility's operations and documentation to verify compliance with these regulations. Other areas have few or no regulations regarding the distribution of oxygen.

If you have any questions regarding oxygen refills or you have difficulty obtaining an oxygen cylinder fill, contact the International DAN office in your region for assistance.

Review Questions

1. The minimum grade of oxygen that is suitable for diving emergencies is:

a. Industrial b. Medical
c. Grade D d. Grade E

2. The potential hazards of breathing high concentrations include: *(Choose all that apply.)*

a. Fire b. Pulmonary Oxygen Toxicity
c. Explosion d. CNS Oxygen Toxicity

3. The potential risks associated with handling oxygen cylinders include: *(Choose all that apply.)*

a. Fire b. Pulmonary Oxygen Toxicity
c. Explosion d. CNS Oxygen Toxicity

4. The DAN Oxygen Provider Card and a prescription are common methods of providing documentation for obtaining oxygen cylinder refills.

a. True b. False

Answers

1. b
2. b, d
3. a, c
4. a

Benefits of Emergency Oxygen for Diving Emergencies

OBJECTIVES

In this chapter you'll learn to

1. **List at least three benefits of providing high oxygen concentrations to an injured diver.**
2. **Describe why an injured diver should receive the highest concentration of oxygen possible.**
3. **State the recommended oxygen concentration that an injured diver should receive.**

KEY TERMS

Barotrauma — Injury of a body part or organ due to changes in pressure.

Basic Life Support ***(BLS)*** — Support or maintenance of life through artificial ventilations or cardiopulmonary resuscitation.

Dehydration — An abnormal depletion of water and other body fluids.

Gradient — A graded difference in physiological activity along an axis *(as of the body or fluid)*.

Hypoxemia — Deficient or reduced oxygenation of the blood.

Inspiration — Inhalation; drawing air into the lungs.

Ischemic — Localized tissue hypoxia due to obstruction or reduced flow of oxygenated blood *(for example, the narrowing of an artery by spasm, illness or injury)*.

Medium — A surrounding or enveloping substance.

Platelet — A round or oval disk found in the blood of vertebrate animals that are involved with blood clotting.

Primary Assessment — Assessment of the Airway, Breathing and Circulation *(pulse)* in an ill or injured person; also known as the ABCs.

As a DAN Oxygen First Aid Provider, your highest priority is basic life support and assisting an injured diver until emergency medical services or other local protocol becomes available. It is also important that you ***do no further harm*** to the injured diver and understand the limits of your training and experience in providing first aid to an injured diver.

Any time a pressure-related dive injury or near-drowning is suspected, 100 percent inspired oxygen should be given following the primary assessment *(ABCs)*. A diver who is having difficulty breathing should receive oxygen. Unresponsive divers are assumed to have respiratory insufficiency and should also receive supplemental oxygen. Oxygen first aid may significantly help a diver experiencing symptoms of a pressure-related diving injury or near-drowning.

The use of emergency oxygen provides a greater chance of complete symptom resolution before recompression treatment. If oxygen first aid is provided, there's also a better chance of being symptom-free after recompression treatment.

The higher the concentration of inhaled oxygen, the faster nitrogen leaves the body.

How does oxygen benefit an injured diver?

When someone has decompression illness *(DCI)*, bubbles that are primarily made up of nitrogen form in the body. When breathing air, nitrogen makes up the majority of the air being inhaled.

If an injured diver inhales 100 percent oxygen, nitrogen is eliminated from the breathing medium. As a result, the inspired oxygen creates a pressure gradient between the lungs, bloodstream and the surrounding tissues that allows for a greater elimination of nitrogen from the tissue. As nitrogen is eliminated from the bloodstream and tissues, more nitrogen is reabsorbed from the bubble into the surrounding tissue and then from the tissue into the bloodstream.

The rate of denitrogenation depends on the difference in partial pressures between the inside of the bubble, the surrounding tissue and the bloodstream. The greater the pressure gradient *(higher concentration of inhaled oxygen)*, the faster nitrogen leaves the body. The use of high concentrations of oxygen may ultimately result in the reduction of bubble size.

All DCI *(arterial gas embolism and decompression sickness)* requires oxygen first aid as quickly as possible. These problems do not necessarily interfere with general oxygen transport except at the site of injury. For example, if the blood supply to the brain is interrupted, the tissue that the blood vessel is feeding will be starved. Permanent damage or death may quickly occur if left unattended. In this instance, high concentration of inspired oxygen is essential. To achieve 100 percent inspired oxygen requires knowledge of the skills and techniques of providing oxygen using a demand inhalator valve.

There are several secondary effects of breathing high partial pressures of oxygen. Circulation in smaller blood vessels can be blocked by nitrogen bubbles, which could cause the tissues to become hypoxic. Breathing high concentrations of oxygen helps oxygenate these hypoxic or ischemic areas.

Oxygen also has an effect on the amount of edema *(or swelling)* produced by the blockage of small blood vessels. This is particularly important in nerve tissue where loss of sensation or function may occur. A reduction in swelling can restore function to the affected nerve tissue.

Blood sludging and the aggregation of platelets occur as bubbles form in the bloodstream. If the injured diver is dehydrated, the sludging effect will be worse. Studies have shown that when oxygen is provided, the amount of sludging is reduced by reducing the number and size of the bubbles. Oral fluids and intravenous fluids also help reverse the effects of dehydration and ensuing sludging.

When the amount of oxygen is decreased in the bloodstream, it is often referred to as hypoxemia. This is seen in near-drownings where the lungs contain water and in heart attacks where there is limited ability to circulate oxygen-enriched blood.

Clearly, from what is known about oxygen and its physiology, immediate oxygen first aid for DCI or near-drowning in the diver will be of considerable benefit.

NOTE: All injured divers must seek an evaluation by a healthcare professional at the nearest medical facility. DAN or DAN-supported Emergency Hotline should be called for an appropriate referral to a physician trained in diving medicine.

Review Questions

1. Providing a high concentration of oxygen to an injured diver provides these benefits: *(Choose all that apply).*

a. May help ease breathing
b. May reduce tissue edema
c. May reduce bubble size
d. Symptoms may be relieved

2. The primary goal of providing the highest concentration of oxygen possible to an injured diver is to facilitate the washout of excess nitrogen.

a. True   b. False

3. It is recommended that injured divers receive ______ % oxygen.

a. 50   b. 75
c. 80   d. 100

Answers

1. a, b, c, d
2. a
3. d

OBJECTIVES

In this chapter you'll learn to

1. List the four components that make up an oxygen delivery system.
2. State the most important feature of an oxygen cylinder.
3. State the purpose of a regulator.
4. Identify the regulator that is able to provide the highest concentration of oxygen to more than one injured diver.
5. Identify the type of oxygen delivery device that will deliver 100 percent oxygen.
6. Identify the constant-flow mask recommended for a second breathing injured diver.
7. Identify the constant-flow mask recommended for performing rescue breathing.

Oxygen Delivery Systems & Components

KEY TERMS

Artificial ventilations — Maintenance of respiratory movements by artificial means. For the general public, this is done most commonly by mouth-to-mouth or mouth-to-mask; also known as rescue breathing and expired air resuscitation *(EAR)*.

Expired air resuscitation *(EAR)* — Involves a rescuer using own expired breath to inflate the lungs and ventilate a non-breathing ill or injured person; also known as rescue breathing and artificial ventilations.

Oronasal — Concerning the mouth and nose.

Rescue Breathing — Providing artificial ventilations or expired air resuscitation during a rescue for a non-breathing ill or injured person.

Oxygen Delivery Systems

The oxygen delivery system consists of an oxygen cylinder, a pressure reducing regulator, a hose and a face mask. While there are many oxygen equipment options, there are some specific guidelines for the use of oxygen equipment for scuba diving injuries.

• ***Oxygen Cylinders*:** Enough oxygen should be available to allow for the continuous delivery of oxygen to an injured diver from the time of injury at the farthest possible dive site to the next level of emergency response. The duration of common portable oxygen cylinders varies based on the size of the oxygen cylinder, the oxygen flow rate and the type of delivery device. However, it is common for a single portable oxygen cylinder to last from 15 minutes to 60 minutes. Non-portable oxygen cylinders can last up to eight hours or more.

• ***Oxygen Regulators*:** There are three common types of regulators for oxygen delivery. One type is a constant-flow style which can deliver a fixed or adjustable flow of oxygen. Unfortunately, oxygen is significantly wasted when constant-flow is used for emergency oxygen delivery. Another style of regulator is the demand regulator. It functions like a scuba regulator and delivers oxygen when the demand valve is activated. The third style of oxygen regulator is the multifunction regulator, which combines the features of both the demand and constant-flow regulators. A multifunction regulator is preferred over the other styles because it will allow a rescuer to provide up to 100 percent oxygen to two injured divers simultaneously and permits various mask options.

• ***Hoses & Tubing:*** Oxygen-safe, clear plastic tubing is provided with certain types of constant-flow masks to connect the mask to the regulator. Since an oxygen demand valve requires approximately 50 psi/ 3.5 Bar, an intermediate pressure hose attaches to the threaded outlets on both the regulator and valve.

• ***Oxygen Mask:*** An oxygen mask is held to the face and permits the inhalation of higher concentrations of oxygen. Oxygen concentrations of 100 percent can be delivered by using a demand valve with oronasal mask. Other oxygen masks vary in the amount of oxygen which can be provided. Common constant flow masks provide from 35 to 75 percent oxygen. For diving injuries, it is recommended that oxygen be delivered by a demand valve and oronasal mask to provide as close to 100 percent inspired oxygen as possible.

For diving injuries, it is recommended that oxygen be delivered by a demand valve and oronasal mask to provide as close to 100 percent inspired oxygen as possible.

Oxygen System Components

Common Oxygen Cylinders

Portable oxygen cylinders come in a variety of sizes. As a DAN Oxygen Provider, your primary concern is capacity. Remember, you should have enough oxygen available to transport an injured diver to nearest appropriate medical facility.

If you conduct shore diving in an area where there is an emergency medical system *(EMS)* in place, you may only need a 15-minute supply. When you dive off a boat close to shore, you may need a one- or two-hour supply. If you are diving far offshore and assistance is hours away, you may want to consider carrying a non-portable oxygen cylinder or multiple portable oxygen cylinders.

Consult your DAN Oxygen Instructor about which cylinder size is most appropriate for your use.

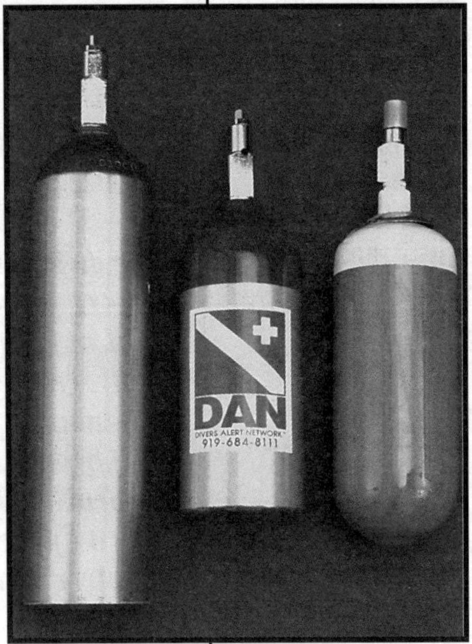

How long a cylinder lasts depends on the consumption of gas. An oxygen cylinder should be changed to a full one when the pressure drops below 200 psi/ 14 bar. However, if only one cylinder is available, it should be used until the oxygen supply is depleted. When using a constant-flow oxygen regulator, it is easy to estimate how long a cylinder will last.

To approximate how long an oxygen cylinder will last using a constant-flow regulator, use this easy formula:

$$\frac{\textit{liter capacity of cylinder}}{\textit{flow rate (lpm)}} = \textit{Time in minutes cylinder will last}$$

Oxygen cylinders are made of different materials and are available in different sizes.

For example, if a cylinder holds 640 liters and the oxygen flow rate is 15 liters per minute, the cylinder will last approximately 43 minutes.

When a diver is using a demand-style regulator, it is more difficult to determine an exact time of supply. The rate at which the oxygen is used will depend on the injured diver's breathing rate and volume. Generally the average oxygen use on a demand valve is equivalent to 8 to 10 liters per minute. Demand-style is preferred because no oxygen is wasted, and usually the oxygen supply lasts longer.

Cylinders are made of either aluminum or steel and are subject to periodic visual and hydrostatic testing. Testing times are generally established by law or regulations, and the requirements vary. Common hydrostatic testing intervals are between two and 10 years. In the USA, the hydrostatic testing requirement is five years

Oxygen cylinders are colored-coded for ease of identification and to minimize the risk of using the contents of a cylinder for an unintended purpose. Common oxygen cylinder color combinations include: green *(United States)*, black with a white shoulder *(Australia, New Zealand, United Kingdom and others)* and white *(Canada and European countries)*. Ask your DAN Oxygen Instructor for the color coding requirements of your region. In addition, oxygen cylinders should be clearly labeled.

The pin indexing system is designed to prevent an oxygen regulator from being used on a cylinder containing another gas.

Pressure Regulators

The pressure regulator reduces the cylinder pressure to a safe working pressure compatible with a demand valve or constant-flow equipment.

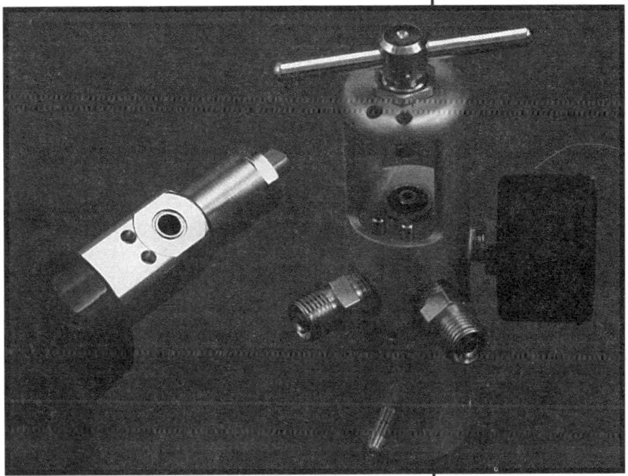

All regulators must have some means of attaching to the oxygen cylinder. Various methods of attachment are available. In some areas, pins engage matching holes on the cylinder valve. This pin-indexed valve is called a CGA 870 medical oxygen valve.

These pins are placed in a specific orientation to prevent an oxygen regulator from being used on a cylinder that may contain another gas. This system is important in locations where there are various gases in use, and each requires its own regulator and cylinder. Pin placement is specific for each gas.

Threaded gas outlet valves are designed to accept regulators intended for medical oxygen use.

In other areas, oxygen cylinders may have threaded gas-outlet valves *(CGA 540 medical oxygen valve and bull-nose valve)* that will accept only regulators intended for medical oxygen use.

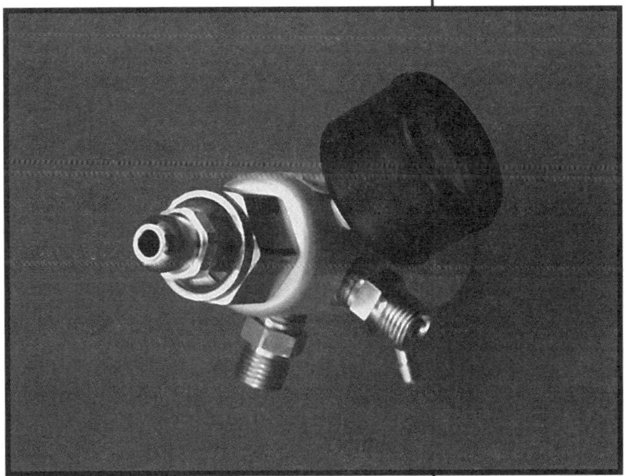

Ask your DAN Oxygen Instructor which connection systems are used in your region for oxygen cylinders and regulators.

Adapters

Oxygen-compatible adapters allow for various regulators be used with other oxygen cylinders.

In some regions, the use of oxygen-compatible adapters allows for various regulators be used with other oxygen cylinders. These adapters provide flexibility when traveling to other areas which may use different cylinders and valves. Adapters also give you the opportunity to use regulators designed for portable oxygen cylinders with non-portable large ones.

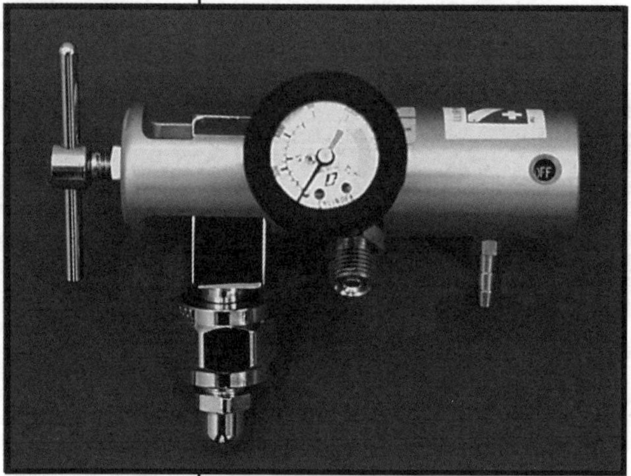

Although oxygen system adapters are available commercially, it is important that they be oxygen-cleaned to minimize the risk of fire and explosion. Avoid homemade adapters and the use of scuba regulators with high concentrations of oxygen.

Avoid homemade adapters and the use of scuba regulators with high concentrations of oxygen.

Flow Meter

The flow meter is an integral part of the pressure regulator and indicates the oxygen flow rate being delivered through the barbed outlet to the constant flow device *(non-rebreather mask or pocket mask)*.

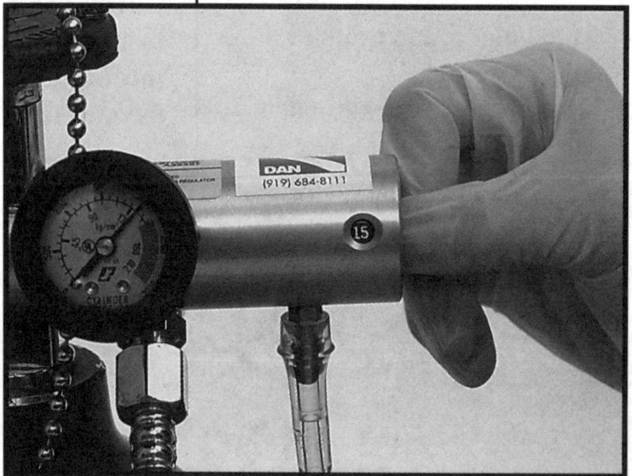

Oxygen flow is measured in liters per minute *(lpm)*. The flow rate is regulated by the control valve on the regulator, with the flow rate indicator window located on the front.

The DAN multi-function regulator is designed to deliver up to 25 lpm. DAN recommends an initial flow rate of 15 lpm when used with either a non-rebreather mask or pocket mask. The goal of oxygen delivery is to deliver the highest concentration of oxygen possible to the injured diver.

The oxygen flow meter indicates the amount of oxygen being delivered to your constant-flow device.

Demand-Style Oxygen Delivery Devices

DAN Demand Inhalator Valve

DAN Oxygen Units contain a demand inhalator valve (similar to a scuba regulator second stage). When an injured diver begins breathing through the mask and a proper seal between the mask and the injured diver's face is maintained, 100 percent oxygen will be inhaled into the injured diver's lungs.

With the demand inhalator valve, oxygen flows only when the injured diver inhales, and the available oxygen supply will often last much longer than with a constant-flow system. The clear Tru-Fit™ mask supplied with the DAN demand inhalator valve is made of a material which provides a good seal for most faces. If the Tru-Fit™ mask does not seal properly, the pocket mask may be substituted. Clear masks allow rescuers to monitor the airway and to watch for indications of breathing and airway obstruction.

Flow-Restricted Oxygen-Powered Ventilator *(FROPV)*

The flow-restricted oxygen-powered ventilator *(FROPV)* is both a demand valve and a manually triggered, oxygen-powered ventilation device. It is designed to assist or control ventilation or to allow a breathing ill or injured person to receive oxygen on demand.

This valve, commonly used by healthcare professionals, has a button *(similar to a scuba regulator purge button)* on top of the valve that controls the flow of oxygen when depressed. This allows the demand resuscitator valve to be used when an ill or injured person is not breathing. It can be a very effective device when used by trained individuals. However, a high degree of training and proficiency is required to properly use the FROPV.

Few dive accidents reported to DAN are of a catastrophic nature. Dive injuries that interrupt breathing are extremely rare.

DAN does not provide training in the use of the FROPV in the Oxygen Provider course for the following reasons:

Oxygen Delivery Device Recommendations

INJURED DIVER
(Breathing)

RECOMMENDED

DAN Demand Inhalator Valve
Non-Rebreather Mask

RECOMMENDED with ADDITIONAL TRAINING

Flow-Restricted Oxygen-Powered Ventilator
Bag Valve Mask

NOT RECOMMENDED

Partial Rebreather
Simple Face Mask
Nasal Cannula

INJURED DIVER
(Non-Breathing)

RECOMMENDED

Pocket Mask

RECOMMENDED with ADDITIONAL TRAINING

Flow-Restricted Oxygen-Powered Ventilator
Bag Valve Mask

Clear masks allow rescuers to monitor the airway and to watch for indications of breathing and airway obstruction.

• Training in the use of the FROPV requires many hours followed by frequent practice to maintain a high degree of proficiency.

Demand inhalator valve with oronasal mask for use with breathing injured divers.

• Studies have shown that skills using the pocket mask with supplemental oxygen have been retained longer by rescuers after long periods of inactivity than the FROPV and other similar devices.

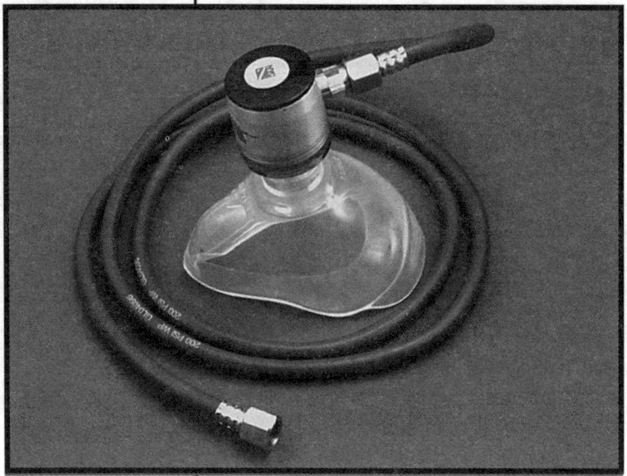

• The use of the pocket mask with supplemental oxygen is much easier to perform than the FROPV with a non-breathing ill or injured person.

DAN realizes the importance of making oxygen first aid training available to the diving public. DAN also recognizes the need to provide accurate information in support of current recommendations in the medical literature. Using an FROPV may not be appropriate for the diver who has not had proper training in its use. Ask your DAN Oxygen Instructor or International DAN (*IDAN*) affiliate for information on other training opportunities.

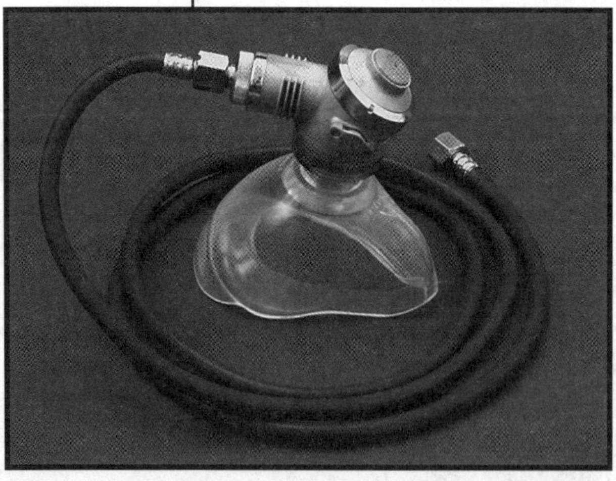

The flow-restricted oxygen-powered ventilator is for use with both breathing and non-breathing injured divers. Additional training is recommended.

Constant-Flow Oxygen Masks

Non-Rebreather Mask

The non-rebreather mask, also known as a high-concentration mask, may be used by the breathing injured diver. This mask is designed to allow an injured diver to inhale oxygen from the reservoir bag positioned below the oronasal mask. The non-rebreather mask consists of a mask with three non-return valves — one on either side of the mask and one separating the mask from the reservoir bag. Oxygen tubing is used to connect the mask to the regulator and is located on the side of the mask where the reservoir bag is attached.

During inhalation, oxygen flows through the mask from the reservoir bag into the injured diver's lungs. The non-return valves on the sides of the mask prevent air from being inhaled which would dilute the oxygen being inhaled.

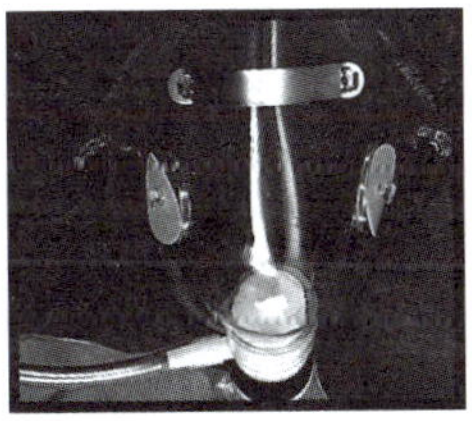

NOTE: Three non-return valves.

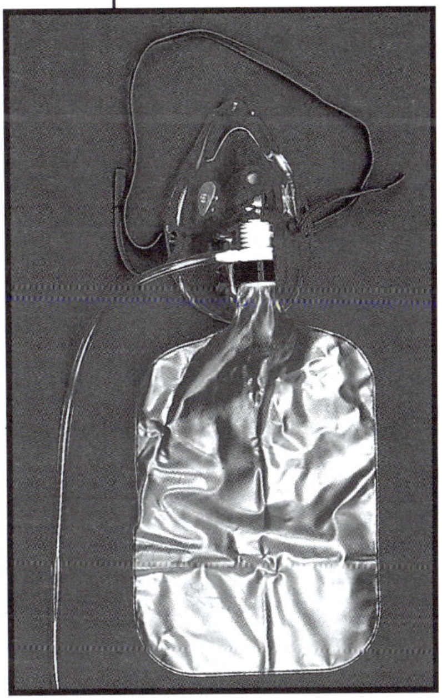

The non-rebreather mask is recommended for the breathing injured diver who does not tolerate the demand inhalator valve, or for a second breathing injured diver.

During exhalation, the one-way valve prevents exhaled air from flowing back into the bag, but it is released to the outside by the one-way valves on the sides of the mask. Additionally, during exhalation, the reservoir bag refills with pure oxygen.

The non-rebreather mask is an effective way of delivering a high concentration of inspired oxygen using the constant-flow feature of the regulator. However, this mask has the disadvantage of requiring a large supply of oxygen because of the constant flow of oxygen. Unless the mask completely seals around the face, air will leak past the mask and valves and dilute the oxygen concentration. This is why this method of oxygen delivery is the second choice after the demand valve for a breathing injured diver.

A non-rebreather mask is recommended for the breathing injured diver who does not tolerate the demand inhalator valve or when there are multiple diving injuries requiring oxygen.

The non-rebreather mask with a good fit, all one-way valves working properly, and proper technique, may deliver inspired oxygen concentrations approaching 90 percent *(65 to 75 percent is considered common).*

Always monitor breathing while providing oxygen first aid using a non-rebreather mask.

Caution: If the oxygen supply to the non-rebreather mask is interrupted and the injured diver has a good seal on the mask, there may be some risk of the injured diver suffocating. Therefore, it is extremely important to never leave an injured diver unattended, and always monitor breathing while providing oxygen first aid using a non-rebreather mask. Remember to always remove any mask prior to turning off the gas supply.

Partial Rebreather Mask

This device combines a simple face mask with a reservoir bag. It is also known as a medium-concentration mask. Like any constant-flow mask, this device will only function properly if it is well-fitted to the face. The flow rate must be higher than 6 liters per minute in order to prevent carbon dioxide buildup. This mask, depending on the flow rate and technique delivers around 60 percent inspired oxygen. This mask is not recommended for use on injured divers because it does not deliver high concentrations of inspired oxygen.

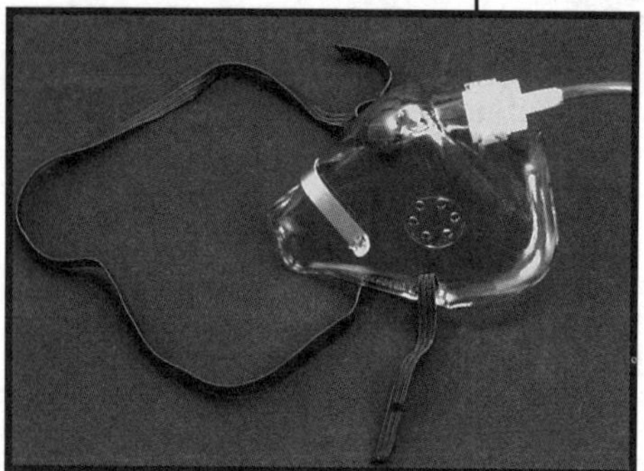

A simple face mask is designed to deliver low to moderate concentrations of oxygen and is not recommended for use with injured divers.

Simple Face Mask

This disposable mask is made of clear plastic and is a common mask found frequently in portable oxygen units. There are small holes in the side of the mask to allow ambient air to mix with oxygen upon inhalation and to allow the exhaled breath to escape. This mask is designed only to deliver low to moderate concentrations of oxygen. According to the manufacturer, the simple face mask may deliver 35 to 60 percent inspired oxygen with high flow rates and exceptional technique. Since this mask delivers moderate concentrations of inspired oxygen, it is not recommended for use with injured divers.

Nasal Cannula

The nasal cannula is a simple tube with two projections *(prongs)* that fit into the nostrils of an ill or injured person. Oxygen flows through the prongs into the nasal passages. Some nasal cannulae have an attached elastic band to hold the device in place. The nasal cannula is most used by patients who require low concentrations of oxygen over long periods of time. This device should not be used for providing oxygen first aid to injured divers because it delivers a very low concentration of inspired oxygen.

Oxygen Masks for Non-Breathing Individuals

There are two options for a rescuer who needs to provide ventilations or rescue breathing for an unresponsive, non-breathing, injured diver. The options are mouth-to-mouth ventilations and mouth-to-mask ventilations. For rescuers who are hesitant to provide mouth-to-mouth ventilations, the mouth-to-mask device employs the same readily available power source *(the rescuer's lungs)* but eliminates direct contact with the injured diver. There are other devices available such as the bag valve mask and flow-restricted oxygen-powered ventilator, but these require more training than is provided in the DAN Oxygen Provider course. Ask your DAN Oxygen Instructor about further training opportunities.

A pocket mask or resuscitation mask is recommended for use with non-breathing injured divers to increase oxygen concentration and prevent disease transmission.

Pocket Mask

The pocket mask is found in DAN's Oxygen Unit and contains a supplemental oxygen inlet. The pocket mask allows the rescuer to provide mouth-to-mask ventilations without direct mouth-to-mouth contact. This device will provide additional oxygen to the non-breathing injured diver if used in conjunction with rescue breathing *(expired air resuscitation or artificial ventilations*) and constant-flow oxygen.

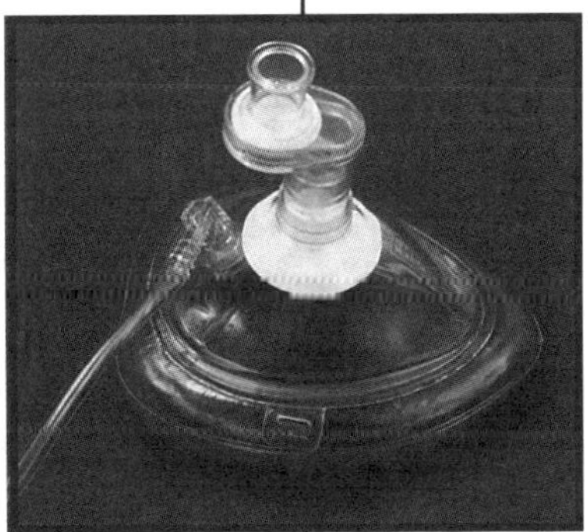

The oronasal mask is made of a clear, flexible material so that it can be collapsed and carried in the pocket. A "chimney" allows the rescuer to blow exhaled air into the injured diver's lungs.

An oxygen inlet on the mask allows oxygen to be delivered to a non-breathing injured diver during mouth-to-mask rescue breathing. Without supplemental oxygen the pocket mask will deliver 16 percent oxygen — the same as mouth-to-mouth ventilations. When supplemental oxygen is used in conjunction with the pocket mask, oxygen concentrations can exceed 50 percent, a substantial improvement over mouth-to-mouth ventilations. Also, the one-way valve when attached to the pocket mask prevents the non-breathing person's exhaled air from blowing back into the rescuer's face, thus reducing the risks of disease transmission.

Bag Valve Mask

The bag valve mask resuscitator is a hand-held device consisting of a self-refilling bag, an oxygen reservoir bag with inlet and a transparent plastic face mask. This device is used on ill or injured persons who are not breathing or to assist someone with weak respirations. It can deliver oxygen concentrations up to 90 percent when attached to an oxygen supply at 15 liters per minute.

The bag valve mask resuscitator is difficult to use effectively. The most common problem is maintaining an effective seal between the face and mask. To properly use this device, the rescuer must be well trained, with skills maintained through frequent practice.

DAN Oxygen Units

DAN's Oxygen Units were specially designed with divers in mind. Each unit is capable of delivering high concentrations of inspired oxygen to injured divers.

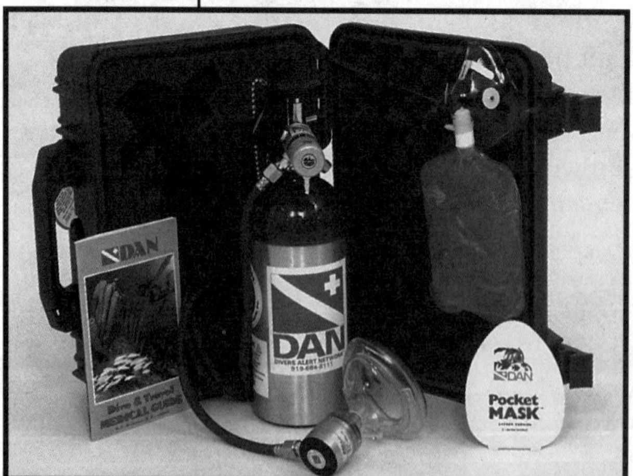

Rescue Pak

The Rescue Pak is an affordable and compact oxygen system that is ideal for areas where emergency medical services *(EMS)* exist nearby or the distance to the nearest medical facility is short. It includes:

- *Multifunction regulator with two-threaded Diameter Indexing Safety System (DISS) outlets, a barbed constant-flow outlet and constant-flow controller (off to 25 lpm) and a pressure gauge*
- *Demand inhalator valve*
- *Non-rebreather mask with clear plastic oxygen supply tubing*
- *Laerdal Pocket Mask™ with oxygen inlet and one-way valve*
- *Oxygen cylinder*
- *Handwheel/wrench with chain*
- *DAN Oxygen Onboard decal*
- *Waterproof hard case*

Standard Oxygen Unit

The Standard Oxygen Unit is a popular choice among divers. This self-contained kit has all the necessary equipment to provide first aid for both breathing and non-breathing injured divers. It includes:

- *Multifunction regulator with two-threaded Diameter Indexing Safety System (DISS) outlets, a barbed constant-flow outlet and constant-flow controller (off to 25 lpm) and a pressure gauge*
- *Demand inhalator valve with clear Tru-Fit™ mask*
- *Non-rebreather mask with clear plastic oxygen supply tubing*
- *Laerdal Pocket Mask™ with oxygen inlet and one-way valve*
- *Oxygen cylinder*
- *Handwheel/wrench with chain*
- *DAN Dive and Travel Medical Guide*
- *DAN Oxygen Onboard decal*
- *Waterproof hard case*

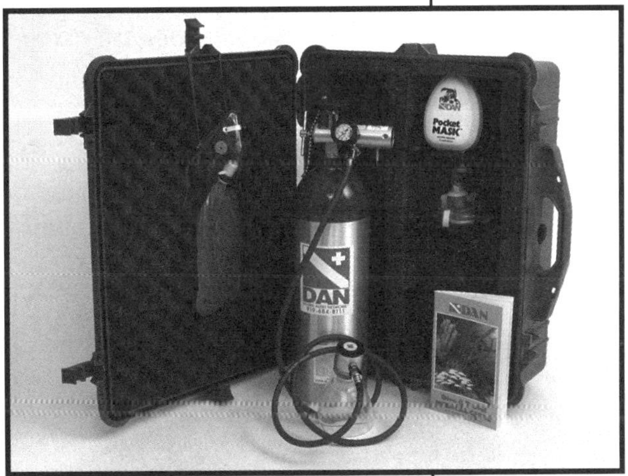

Dual Cylinder Unit

DAN's Dual Cylinder Unit is ideal for offshore diving or for divers who desire a greater oxygen supply. It includes:

- *Multifunction regulator with two-threaded Diameter Indexing Safety System (DISS) threaded outlets, a barbed constant-flow outlet and constant-flow controller (off to 25 lpm) and a pressure gauge*

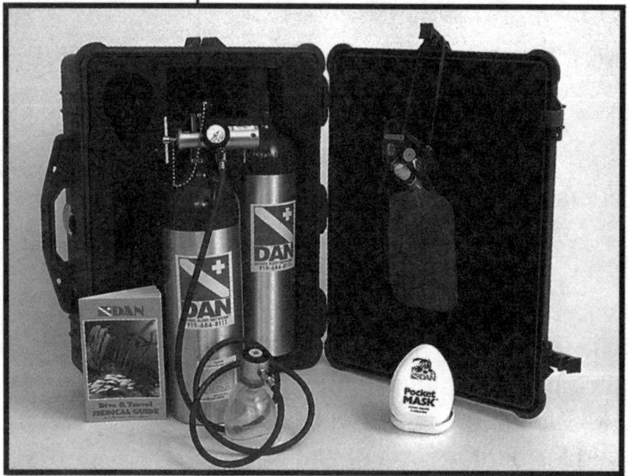

- *Demand inhalator valve with clear Tru-Fit™ mask*
- *Non-rebreather mask with clear plastic oxygen supply tubing*
- *Laerdal Pocket Mask™ with supplemental oxygen inlet*
- *Two oxygen cylinders*
- *Handwheel/wrench with chain*
- *DAN Dive and Travel Medical Guide*
- *DAN Oxygen Onboard decal*
- *Waterproof hard case*

Mini-Unit

DAN's Mini-Unit, which does not include an oxygen cylinder, is compact and allows the diver to transport the equipment to the dive site hassle-free when oxygen cylinders are available locally. It fits in the overhead compartment or under the seat of an airplane or in most dive bags for travel. It includes:

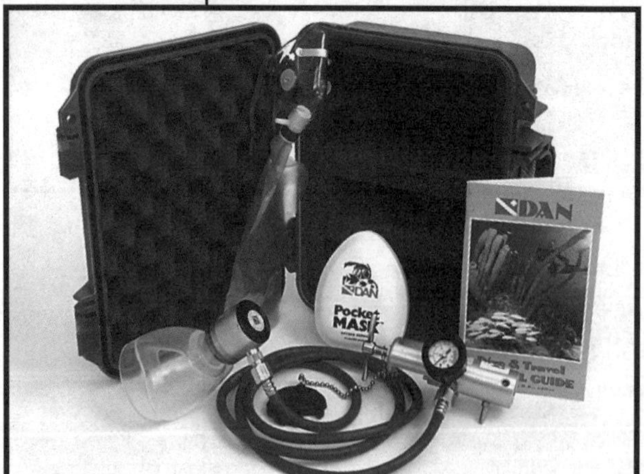

- *Multifunction regulator with two-threaded Diameter*

Indexing Safety System (DISS) threaded outlets, a barbed constant-flow outlet and constant-flow controller (off to 25 lpm) and a pressure gauge

- *Demand inhalator valve with clear Tru-Fit™ mask*
- *Non-rebreather-mask with clear plastic oxygen supply tubing*
- *Laerdal Pocket Mask™ with supplemental oxygen inlet*
- *Handwheel/wrench with chain*
- *DAN Dive and Travel Medical Guide*
- *DAN Oxygen Onboard decal*
- *Waterproof hard casc*

Charter Boat Unit

DAN's Charter Boat Unit contains the same components as DAN's Mini-Unit except the multifunction regulator has a CGA-540 threaded connection system designed for large *(non-portable)* oxygen cylinders.
It includes:

- *Multifunction regulator with two-threaded Diameter Indexing Safety System (DISS) threaded outlets, a barbed constant-flow outlet and constant-flow controller (off to 25 lpm) and a pressure gauge*
- *Demand inhalator valve with clear Tru-Fit™ mask*
- *Non-rebreather mask with clear plastic oxygen supply tubing*
- *Laerdal Pocket Mask™ with supplemental oxygen inlet*

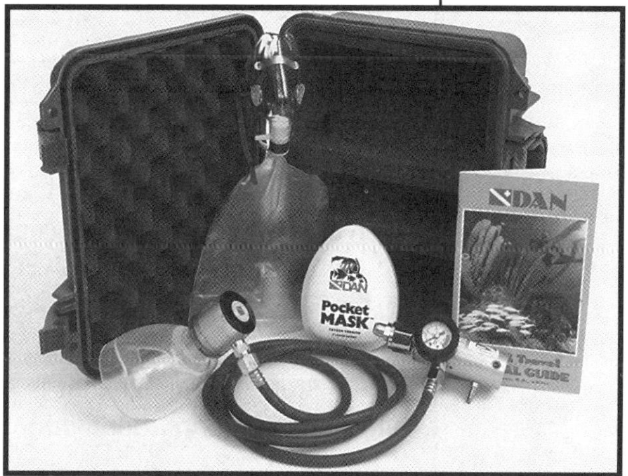

- *Handwheel/ wrench with chain*
- *DAN Dive and Travel Medical Guide*
- *DAN Oxygen Onboard decal*
- *Waterproof hard case*

Review Questions

1. A oxygen delivery system consists of: *(Choose all that apply).*

a. Oxygen cylinder
b. Oxygen delivery device or mask
c. Hoses or tubing
d. Oxygen regulator

2. The most important feature in deciding which oxygen cylinder you should use is:

a. Material
b. Valve
c. Capacity or volume
d. Testing intervals

3. The purpose of a regulator is to reduce high pressure oxygen to an intermediate pressure for delivery by a mask.

a. True
b. False

4. Match the following:

Non-rebreather mask _______
Multifunction regulator _______
Pocket mask _______
Demand inhalator valve _______

a. Will deliver 100 percent oxygen.
b. Will provide the highest concentration of oxygen to more than one injured diver
c. Constant-flow mask that is recommended for performing rescue breathing
d. Constant-flow mask that is recommended for more than one breathing injured diver.

Answers

1. a, b, c, d
2. c
3. a
4. d, b, c, a

Oxygen Provider Skills Development

Scene Safety Assessment

Follow these simple steps to perform a Scene Safety Assessment

Remember S-A-V-E

S STOP

- Stop.
- Think.
- Act.
- Locate barriers & Oxygen Unit.

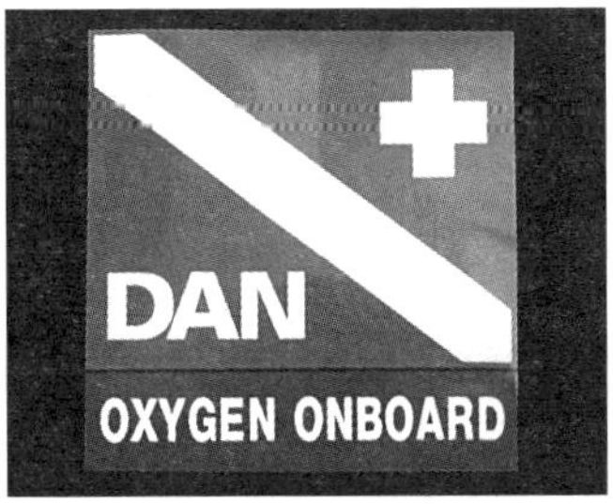

A ASSESS Scene

- Is diving equipment secure?
- Have divers been recalled?
- Any other hazards present?

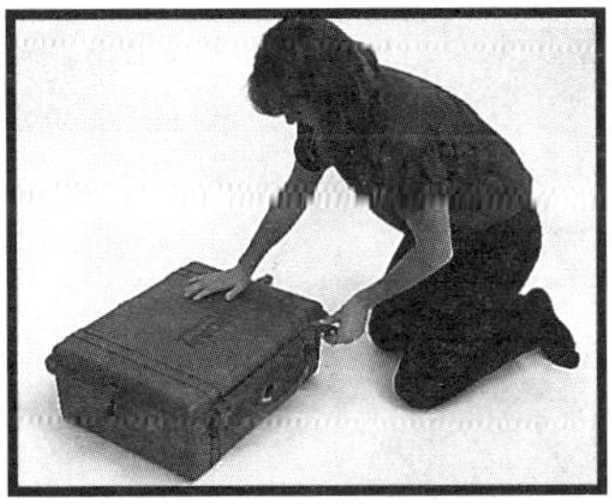

V VENTILATION for Oxygen Adequate

- Smoking materials extinguished?
- Avoid oils, grease and other contamination.
- Avoid enclosed areas.

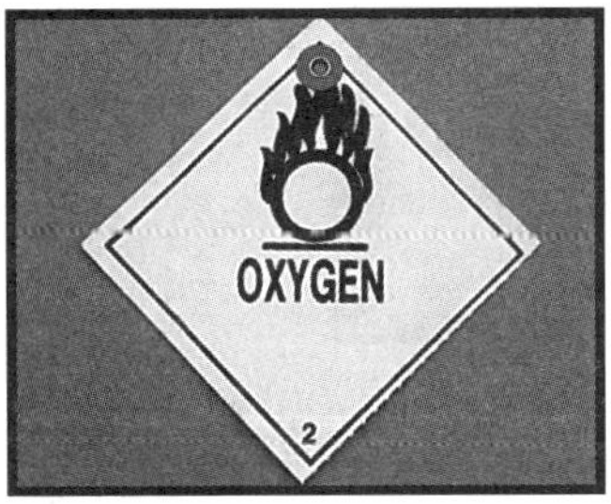

E EXPOSURE Protection

- Use barriers such as gloves and mouth-to-mask devices.

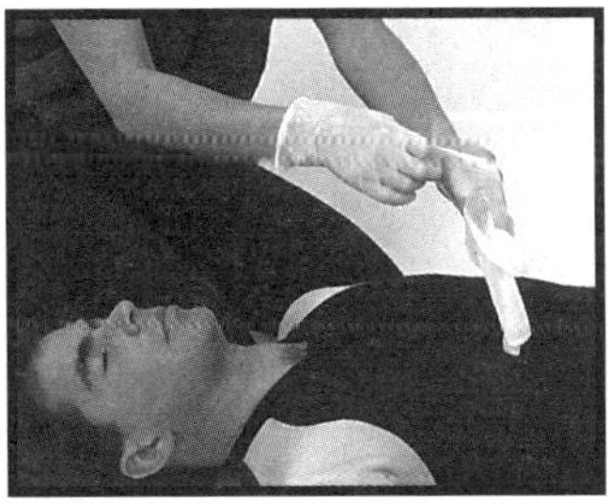

REMEMBER	***AVOID***
◆ SAVE yourself first	◆ Rushing to help without thinking first
◆ Use barrier devices	◆ Contact with blood and other bodily fluids

OBJECTIVES

In this chapter you'll learn to:

1. **Perform a scene safety assessment for oxygen use.**
2. **List the steps in performing a scene safety assessment.**
3. **Assess the Airway, Breathing and Circulation (ABCs) of an injured diver.**
4. **Establish and maintain the Airway and Breathing *(perform Rescue Breathing)* of an injured diver in both the one- and two-rescuer position.**
5. **Provide oxygen to a responsive breathing injured diver using the demand inhalator valve and Tru-Fit™ mask.**
6. **Provide oxygen to an unresponsive breath ing injured diver using the non-rebreather mask.**
7. **Establish and maintain the Airway and Breathing *(perform Rescue Breathing)* of an injured diver with supplemental oxygen using a pocket mask.**
8. **Provide oxygen simultaneously to two injured divers.**
9. **Assemble and disassemble the DAN Oxygen Unit.**

Basic Life Support: *Assessment*

Follow these simple steps to assess
AIRWAY, BREATHING & CIRCULATION *(ABCs)*

Remember S-A-V-E

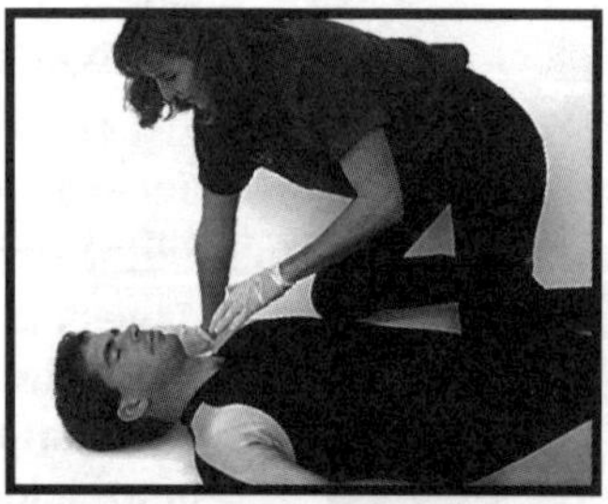

Tap and shout.

ASSESS RESPONSIVENESS

- Tap on the shoulder.
- Shout "Are you OK.?"
- Identify yourself.
- If unresponsive, activate emergency medical services (EMS) and call for help.

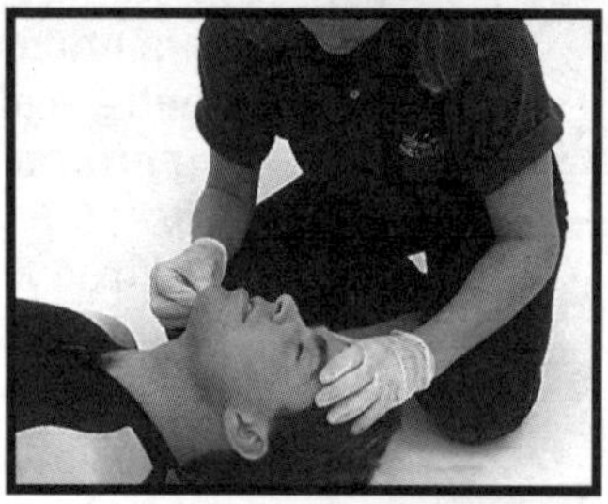

Open Airway.

OPEN AIRWAY

- Use head-tilt, chin-lift method if head, neck or spine injury is not suspected.
- Place one hand on injured diver's forehead.
- Place other hand on the chin and lift jaw.

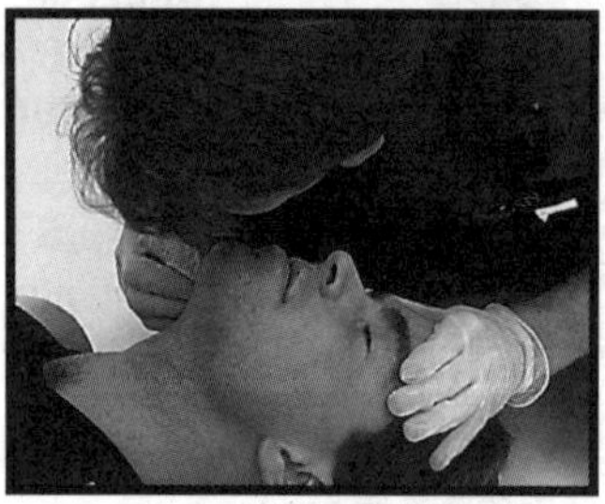

Assess Breathing.

ASSESS BREATHING

- Look, listen and feel for breathing for up to 10 seconds.
- Look for the chest to rise and fall.
- Listen for breathing sounds.
- Feel for breathing against your skin.

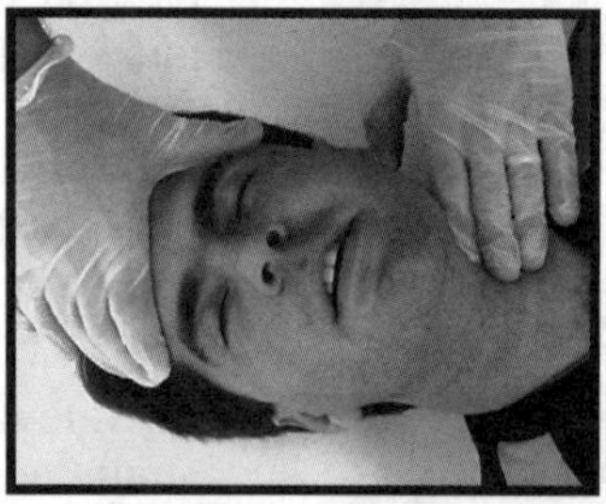

Assess Circulation *(Check Pulse)*.

ASSESS CIRCULATION

- Locate pulse.
- Find Adam's apple with two or three fingers.
- Slide fingers into the groove of neck closest to you.
- Check pulse for up to 10 seconds.

REMEMBER

◆ Keep airway open at all times
◆ If patient is responsive, breathing and circulation are assured

AVOID

◆ Neck lift to open airway
◆ Using your thumb to check pulse

Basic Life Support: *Procedures & Techniques*

Follow these simple steps to perform
RESCUE BREATHING

Remember S-A-V-E

ASSESS RESPONSIVENESS

- If unresponsive, activate emergency medical services (EMS) and call for help.

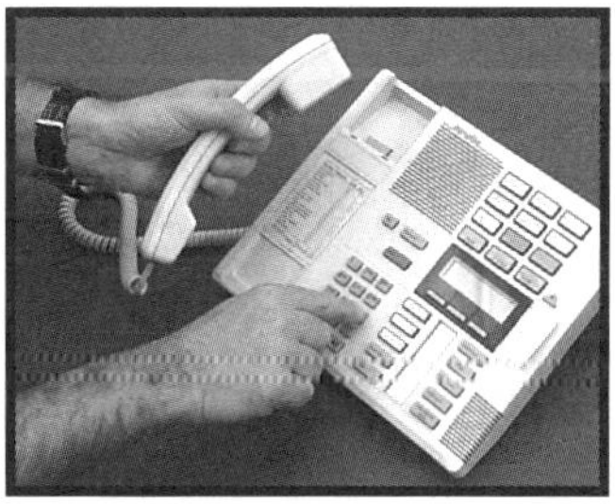

If not responsive, call for help.

OPEN AIRWAY

- Using head-tilt chin-lift method.

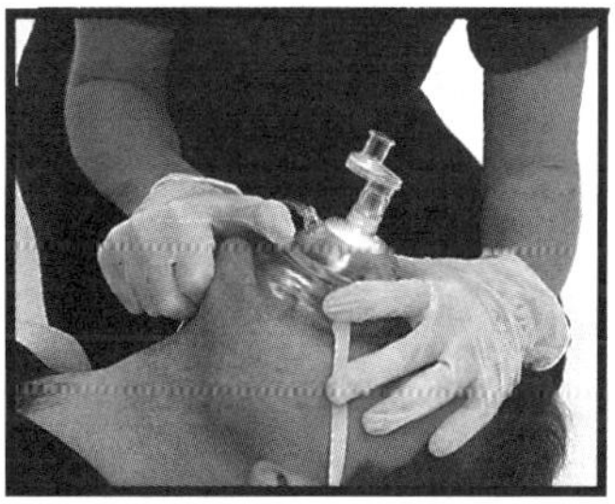

Use barriers when performing Rescue Breathing.

ASSESS BREATHING

- If not breathing, maintain airway and place pocket mask on injured diver's face.
- Provide two slow breaths of 1.5 to 2 seconds in duration.
- Look for the chest to rise and fall.

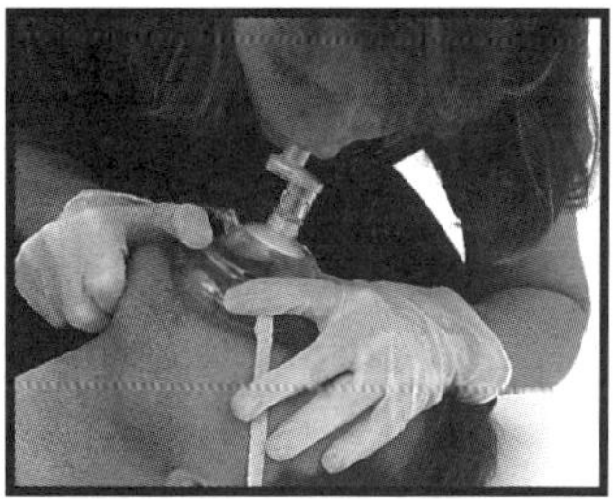

Give two slow breaths *(1.5-2 seconds' duration).*

ASSESS CIRCULATION

- If there's a pulse, give one breath every 5 seconds
- If no pulse, begin CPR.

Note: CPR may be taught as a module with this program.

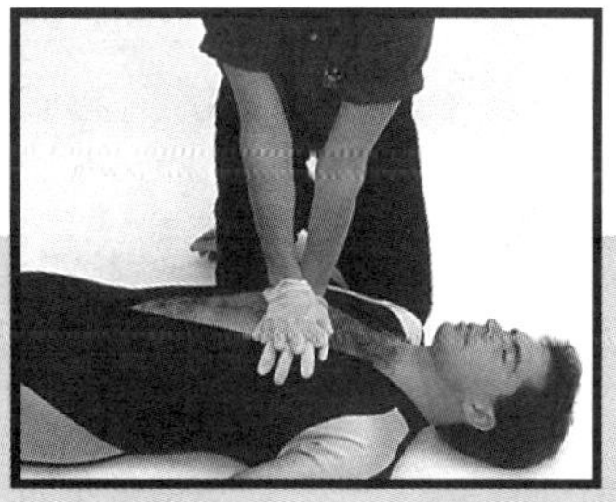

If no pulse, begin CPR.

REMEMBER

◆ Provide slow, full, rescue breaths

◆ If vomit or other fluids are visible in the airway, turn the diver on the side and clear the airway

◆ To check pulse regularly

◆ To maintain an open airway

◆ If rescue breaths are unsuccessful, reposition the airway and reattempt rescue breathing

AVOID

◆ Forceful, rapid rescue breaths

◆ Contact with blood and other bodily fluids

Oxygen Provider Skills: *Demand Inhalator Valve*

Follow these simple steps to provide oxygen to a responsive or unresponsive breathing injured diver with the Demand Inhalator Valve. This is the preferred method of providing emergency oxygen to any breathing injured diver.

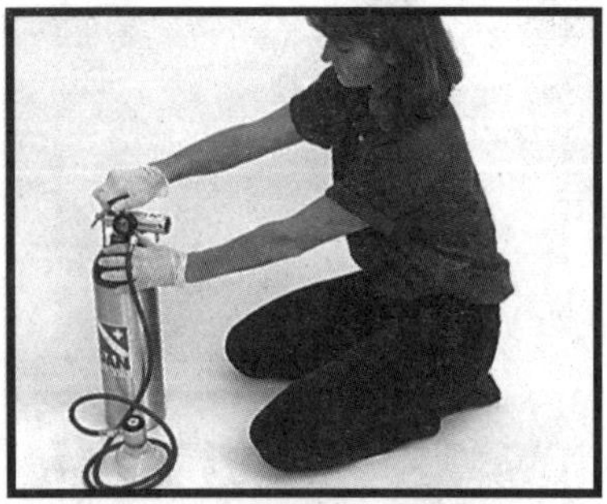

Deploy the oxygen unit.

Remember S-A-V-E

ASSURE AIRWAY, BREATHING & CIRCULATION

INFORM THE INJURED DIVER THAT OXYGEN MAY HELP

- State: *"This is oxygen and it may make you feel better. May I help you?"*
- If the injured diver is unresponsive, permission to help is assumed.

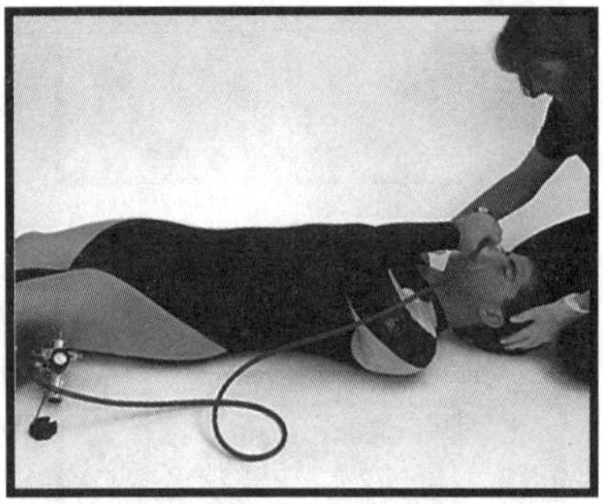

Demand inhalator valve may be used for the responsive breathing injured diver.

DEPLOY THE OXYGEN UNIT

- Open cylinder valve with one complete turn.
- Check cylinder pressure.
- Assure that there are no leaks in the system.
- Constant-flow setting should be in "Off" position.
- Take breath and exhale away from demand valve.

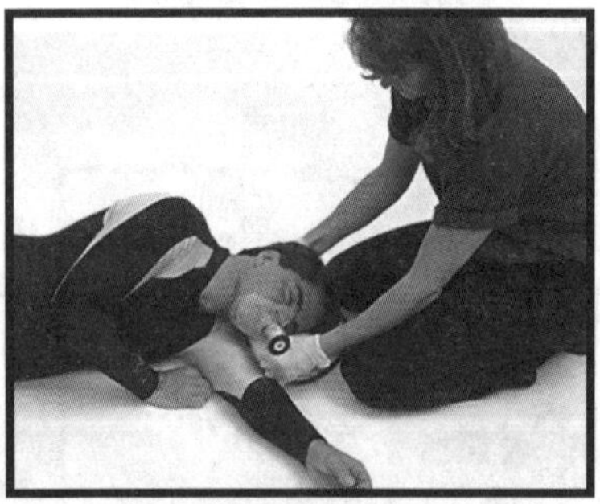

Demand inhalator valve also may be used for the unresponsive breathing injured diver.

PLACE THE MASK OVER THE INJURED DIVER'S MOUTH AND NOSE

- Check the mask for any leaks around injured diver's face.

INSTRUCT THE INJURED DIVER TO BREATHE NORMALLY FROM THE MASK

- Reassure and comfort injured diver.

INSTRUCT THE INJURED DIVER TO HOLD THE MASK TO HELP MAINTAIN A TIGHT SEAL

MONITOR THE INJURED DIVER AND OXYGEN PRESSURE GAUGE

- Listen for the demand inhalator valve to open during inspiration.
- Observe mask fogging during exhalation and clearing with inhalation.
- Watch the chest rise during inhalation and fall with exhalation.

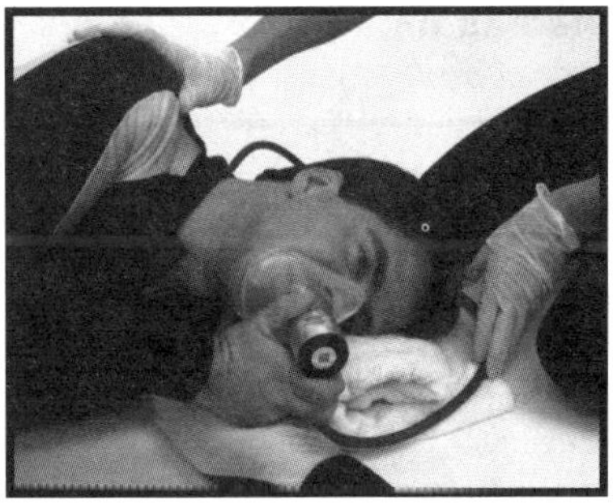

Always reassure and comfort the injured diver.

ACTIVATE EMERGENCY ACTION PLAN

- Call EMS or other appropriate medical facility.
- Contact DAN for consultation and coordination of hyperbaric treatment.

REMEMBER

◆ Turn oxygen cylinder valves on slowly
◆ Call EMS or other appropriate medical facility
◆ Contact DAN for consultation and coordination of hyperbaric treatment
◆ At no time should oxygen first aid be used in lieu of definitive care by a trained healthcare provider

AVOID

◆ Looking at the pressure gauge when turning on cylinder
◆ Exhaling into the demand valve when checking the unit

Oxygen Provider Skills: *Non-Rebreather Mask*

Follow these simple steps to provide oxygen to a responsive or unresponsive breathing injured diver with the non-rebreather mask. The non-rebreather mask is ideal when you have two injured divers or if an injured diver who will not tolerate the demand inhalator valve.

Attach the oxygen tubing to the barbed constant-flow outlet and set the flow rate to 15 lpm initially.

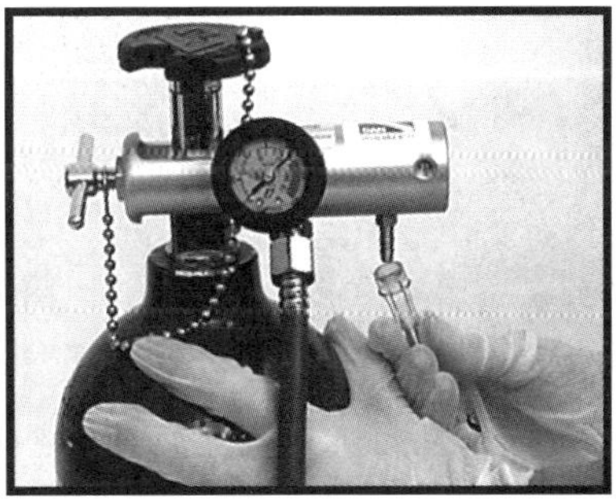

Remember S-A-V-E

ASSURE AIRWAY, BREATHING & CIRCULATION

INFORM THE INJURED DIVER THAT OXYGEN MAY HELP AND ASK PERMISSION TO HELP

DEPLOY THE OXYGEN UNIT

Remember to prime the reservoir bag on the non-rebreather mask.

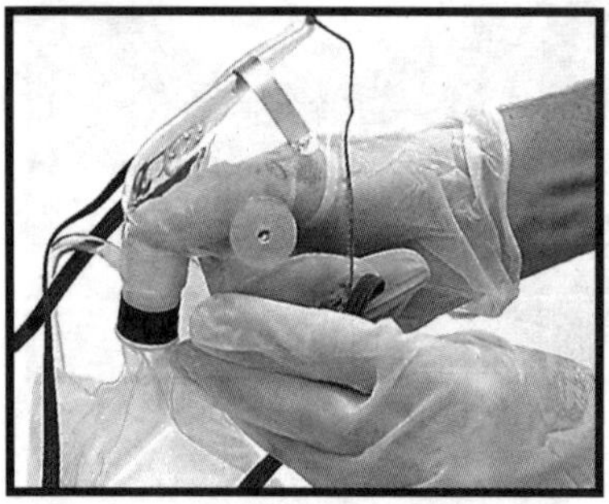

REMOVE NON-REBREATHER MASK FROM BAG

- Stretch oxygen tubing to avoid kinks.
- Attach oxygen tubing to barbed constant flow outlet on multifunction regulator.

SET CONSTANT-FLOW CONTROL TO 15 LITERS PER MINUTE *(lpm)*

PRIME MASK RESERVOIR BAG

- Place a thumb or finger inside the nosepiece, closing the non-return valve, until the reservoir bag fully inflates.

Secure the mask and check for leaks.

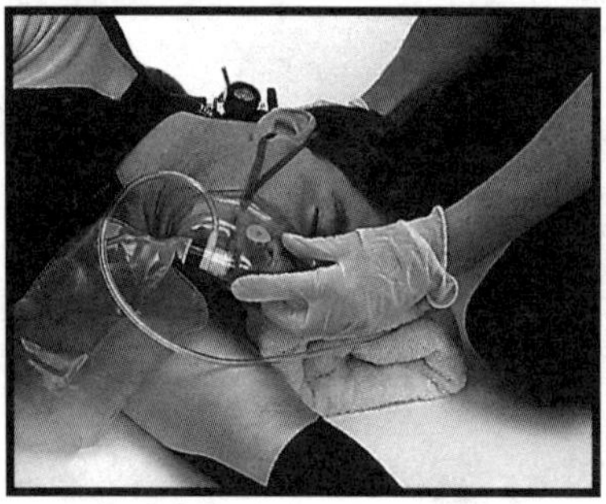

PLACE THE MASK OVER THE INJURED DIVER'S MOUTH AND NOSE

- Check the mask for any leaks around injured diver's face.
- Adjust the elastic band around head to hold the mask in place.
- Squeeze the metal clip over the nose to improve the seal and prevent leakage of oxygen around the mask.

If reservoir bag deflates, increase flow rate to 25 lpm.

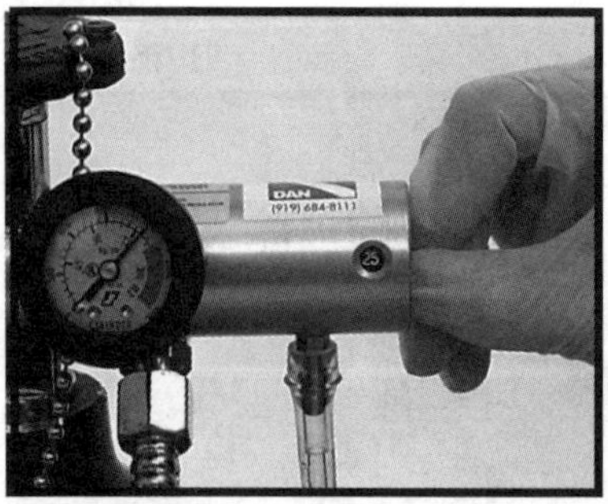

INSTRUCT THE INJURED DIVER TO BREATHE NORMALLY

- Assure reservoir bag remains inflated.
- If not, increase flow rate to 25 lpm.
- Reassure and comfort injured diver.

PLACE THE INJURED DIVER IN PROPER POSITION

IF RESPONSIVE, INSTRUCT THE INJURED DIVER TO HOLD MASK TO MAINTAIN A TIGHT SEAL

MONITOR THE INJURED DIVER AND THE OXYGEN SYSTEM PRESSURE GAUGE

- Look for the reservoir bag to slightly inflate and deflate and for movement of the non-return valves.
- Observe mask fogging during exhalation and clearing with inhalation.
- Watch the chest rise during inhalation and fall with exhalation.

ACTIVATE EMERGENCY ACTION PLAN

- Call EMS or other appropriate medical facility.
- Contact DAN for consultation and coordination of hyperbaric treatment.

REMEMBER

◆ Prime reservoir bag
◆ Turn oxygen cylinder valves on slowly
◆ Call EMS or other appropriate medical facility
◆ Contact DAN for consultation and coordination of hyperbaric treatment
◆ At no time should oxygen first aid be used in lieu of definitive care by a trained healthcare provider

AVOID

◆ Looking at the pressure gauge when turning on cylinder
◆ Allowing the reservoir bag to completely deflate

Oxygen Provider Skills: *Pocket Mask*

Follow these simple steps to provide oxygen to an unresponsive non-breathing injured diver using the pocket mask. The use of the pocket mask with supplemental oxygen is the preferred method of providing oxygen to a non-breathing injured diver for the single rescuer. IMPORTANT NOTE: Do not delay rescue breathing in order to obtain oxygen.

Remember S-A-V-E

ASSURE AIRWAY, BREATHING & CIRCULATION

ACTIVATE EMERGENCY ACTION PLAN

INFORM THE INJURED DIVER THAT OXYGEN MAY HELP AND ASK PERMISSION TO HELP

DEPLOY THE OXYGEN UNIT

PREPARE THE POCKET MASK

Attach the one-way valve to the pocket mask.

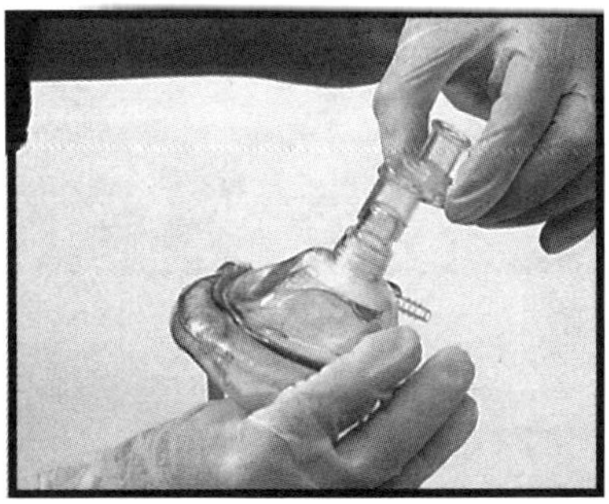

Attach oxygen tubing to oxygen inlet on the pocket mask.

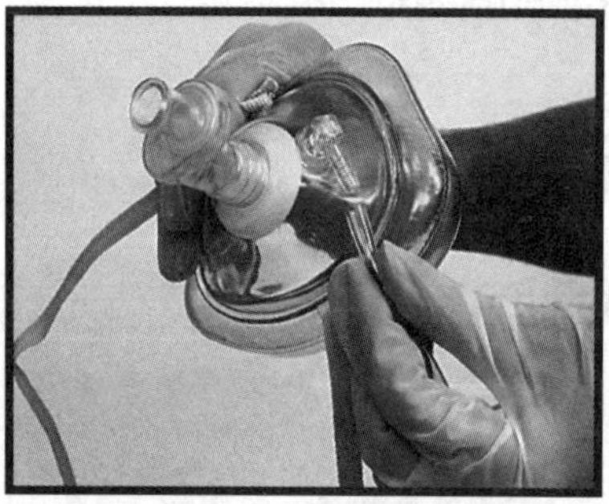

- Remove mask from case.
- Attach one-way valve.
- Remove oxygen tubing from the non-rebreather mask.
- Attach oxygen tubing on the barbed constant-flow outlet on the multifunction regulator and the oxygen inlet on the pocket mask.
- Set constant-flow control to 15 liters per minute (lpm).
- Listen for flow of oxygen.

PLACE THE POCKET MASK OVER THE INJURED DIVER'S MOUTH AND NOSE

- Adjust the elastic band around head to hold the mask in place.

Set constant-flow control to 15 lpm and listen for the flow of oxygen.

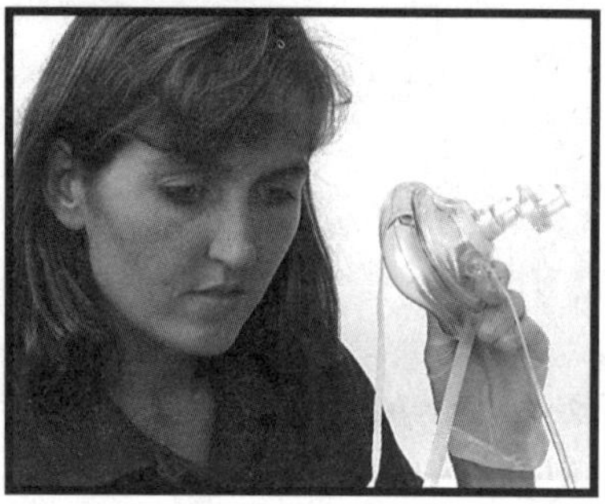

OPEN AIRWAY USING HEAD-TILT CHIN-LIFT METHOD

ASSESS BREATHING

- Look, listen and feel for breathing for up to 10 seconds.
- Look for the chest to rise and fall and for condensation on the inside of the mask.
- Listen for breathing sounds.
- If not breathing, perform rescue breathing.
- Maintain open airway and lift the chin up to the mask.
- Take deep breath.
- Provide two slow breaths of 1.5 to 2 seconds in duration.
- Watch for the chest to rise and fall

If not breathing, provide rescue breaths with supple-mental oxygen.

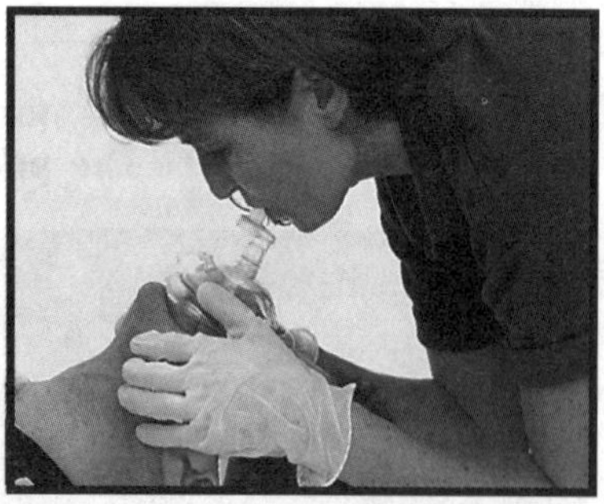

ASSESS CIRCULATION

- Locate pulse.
- Find Adam's apple with two or three fingers.
- Slide fingers into the closest neck groove to you.
- Check pulse for up to 10 seconds.
- If there's a pulse, give one breath every 5 seconds.
- If no pulse, begin CPR.

REMEMBER

- Do not delay rescue breathing in order to obtain oxygen
- Maintain an open airway
- If the injured diver begins breathing the pocket mask may remain in place and oxygen flow continued until breathing is well established
- Once breathing is well established, the demand inhalator valve or non-rebreather mask may replace the pocket mask to provide the injured diver with a higher concentration of oxygen
- Prepare and use appropriate barriers

AVOID

- Forceful or rapid rescue breaths
- Contact with blood or other bodily fluids

Oxygen Provider Skills: *Oxygen Equipment Assembly and Disassembly*

Follow these simple steps to assemble and disassemble the DAN Oxygen Unit.

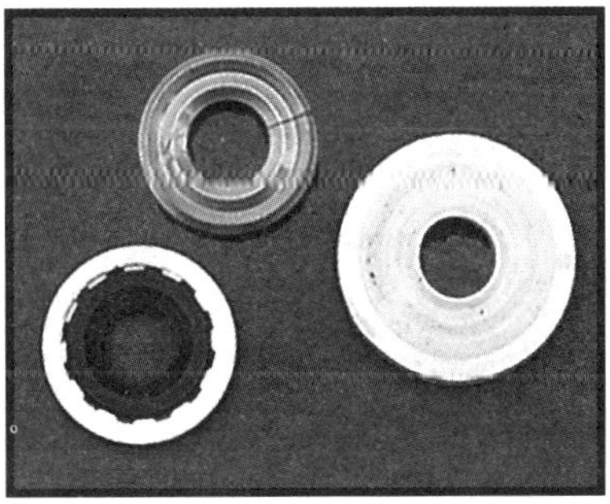

These various types of washers create a seal between the regulators and the cylinders.

ASSURE OXYGEN UNIT IS DEPRESSURIZED

- Open constant-flow control.
- Check pressure gauge.

REMOVE MULTIFUNCTION REGULATOR FROM THE OXYGEN CYLINDER VALVE

- Secure oxygen cylinder.

REMOVE OXYGEN WASHER FROM MULTIFUNCTION REGULATOR

- Note: Washer is different from standard scuba O-ring.

Be careful to avoid contaminating components of the oxygen system.

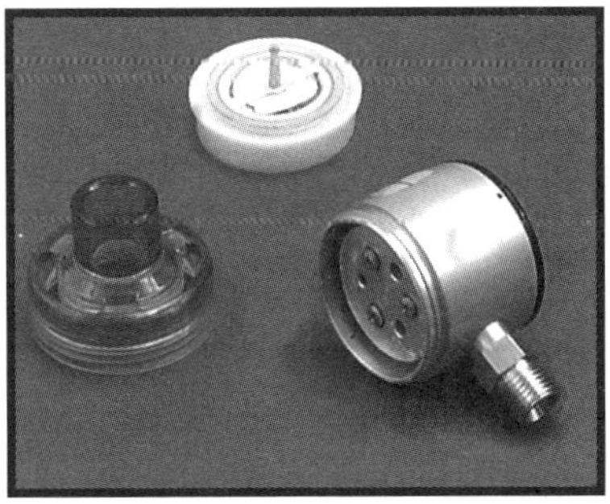

REMOVE OXYGEN HOSE FROM MULTIFUNCTION REGULATOR

- If the fitting is too tight, use handwheel/wrench to unscrew the hose.
- Note: Check valves assure oxygen does not flow from DISS (demand) ports.

REMOVE OXYGEN HOSE FROM DEMAND INHALATOR VALVE

• Note: Both ends of the oxygen hose are identical.

UNSCREW THE PLASTIC MASK ADAPTER FROM THE DEMAND INHALATOR VALVE

REMOVE INHALATION / EXHALATION ASSEMBLY

TO ASSEMBLE: REPEAT STEPS IN REVERSE

REMEMBER

◆ Depressurize oxygen system before disassembly

◆ Check the system for leaks

◆ Both ends of the oxygen hose are identical

◆ Handwheel/wrench is used to loosen and not tighten hoses

◆ Check valves are to assure oxygen does not leak from the system when demand valves are not used

AVOID

◆ Cross-threading the connections on the hoses and demand inhalator valve's plastic mask adapter

◆ Contamination of oxygen components

Recommendations for Oxygen Use

Check the Oxygen Unit's contents and cylinder pressure well before every dive outing.

Keep the cylinder completely filled with oxygen at all times.

The emergency oxygen unit should remain in the case, fully assembled, and turned off. This allows for rapid deployment of the unit.

Never store an oxygen system with the valve open and/or the regulator pressurized. The oxygen may be drained if there is a leak that goes undetected.

Always store the oxygen cylinder securely in its protective, waterproof case in order to reduce the likelihood of damage to component parts and prevent exposure to the corrosive properties of sea water.

Extra cylinders, washers and masks are strongly recommended for extended delivery times and for assisting several injured divers.

The oxygen unit should be professionally serviced once every two years by a trained and authorized service representative or the oxygen equipment manufacturer. Never allow oxygen equipment to come in contact with any grease or oils; they can cause an explosion or fire.

When turning an oxygen cylinder valve on, always turn it slowly to allow the system to pressurize. This will reduce the possibility of an oxygen fire if combustible contaminants have been introduced into the system. Once the system is pressurized, open the valve at least one full turn.

Oxygen masks must be cleaned thoroughly. Follow the recommendations of your DAN Oxygen Instructor. One method is to soak the masks in a mild bleach solution *(10 percent in water)*, rinse with fresh water, and thoroughly dry after each use. Harsh detergents or other chemical cleaning agents may deteriorate the masks and cause skin irritations when they come in contact with the injured diver's skin. Other recommendations include chlorheridine and alcohol.

OBJECTIVES

In this chapter you'll learn to:

1. **List the steps in performing a pre-dive check of your oxygen unit.**
2. **Store your oxygen unit.**
3. **List the recommendations for oxygen unit service intervals.**
4. **List the recommendations for oxygen unit and mask cleaning.**
5. **Identify the position in which an injured diver should be placed.**
6. **Identify the type of fluids recommended for injured divers.**
7. **State where an injured diver should be transported following an injury.**

Recommendations for Oxygen Providers Basic Life Support

Cardiopulmonary resuscitation (CPR) should be learned before you are trained to provide emergency oxygen. The CPR-trained diver and is unlikely to use the skill for an injured diver and is more likely to use it in the course of everyday life. Proficiency in CPR is not difficult, but it does require training and practice under the supervision of a qualified instructor. This manual is not intended as a resource in learning cardiopulmonary resuscitation.

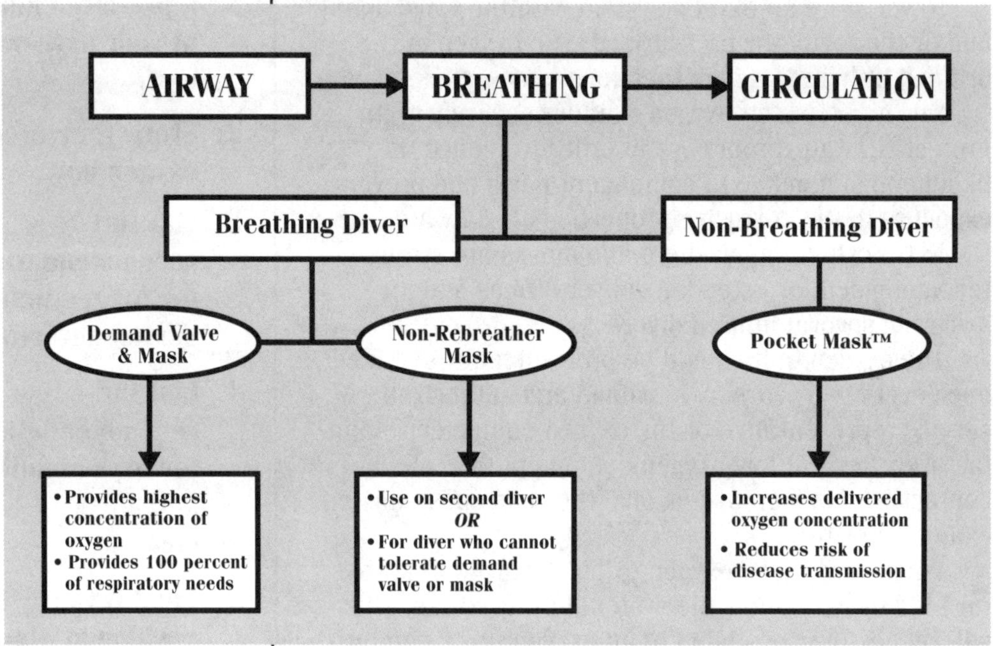

Dive Accident Positioning

An injured diver should be placed in a proper position. The diver's responsiveness and breathing status determine the best position for providing basic life support and oxygen.

- ***RESPONSIVE, BREATHING INJURED DIVER***

This is the supine position.

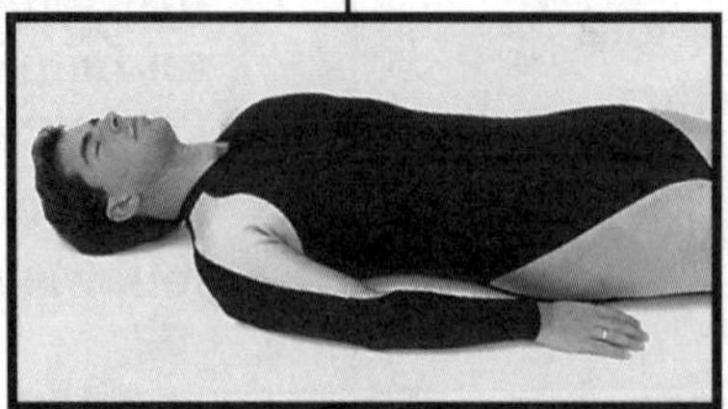

If an injured diver is responsive and fully alert, he/she may be placed in any comfortable horizontal position such as the supine position *(lying flat on the back)* or the recovery position, also known as the lateral recumbent position, where the person is placed on the side with head supported at a low angle and the upper leg bent at the knee.

It is important not to obstruct blood flow by crossing the injured diver's arms or legs. Inert gas elimination is still occurring, and obstructed blood flow to an extremity may interfere with efficient offgassing.

This is the recovery, or lateral recumbent position.

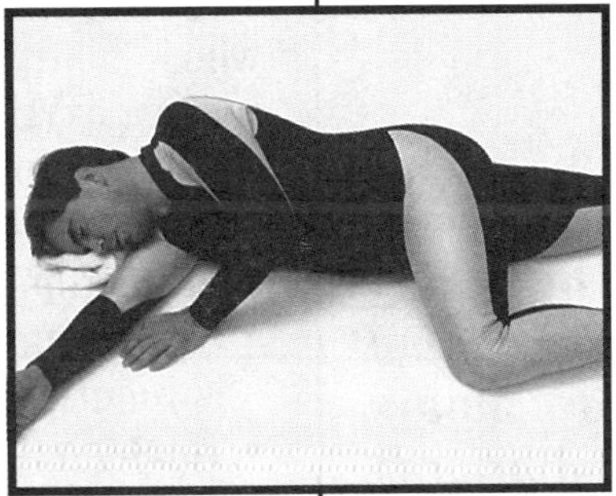

• *UNRESPONSIVE, BREATHING INJURED DIVER*

An injured diver who is unresponsive but breathing should be placed in the lateral recumbent position. This minimizes the risk of airway obstruction by the tongue for the injured diver with a reduced conscious level. In addition, if vomiting occurs in this position, gravity will help keep the airway clear. In this situation, the Oxygen Provider should remove the mask, clear the airway, and reassess the ABCs before resuming oxygen first aid.

Be sure to clear the airway of any obstruction or vomitus.

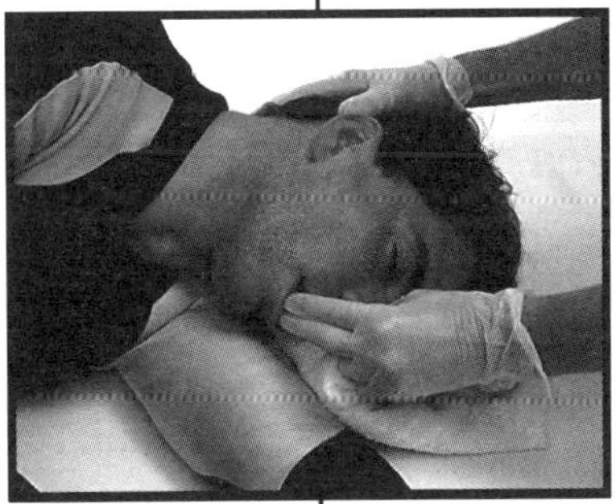

• *UNRESPONSIVE, NON-BREATHING INJURED DIVER*

When an injured diver is not breathing, the diver must be placed on the back *(supine)* so that either rescue breathing *(artificial ventilations or expired air resuscitation) or* CPR may be initiated. Vomiting in this position is extremely dangerous, and if it occurs, the injured diver should be quickly turned to the side until the airway is cleared so that aspiration *(inhaling)* of vomitus does not occur. Once the airway is cleared, resuscitation efforts can resume, with the diver in the supine position.

When turning the injured diver, protect the head, neck and spine.

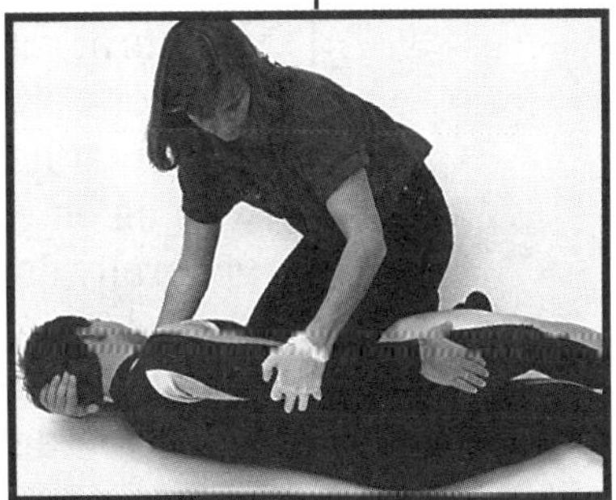

• *TURNING THE INJURED DIVER*

Care should be taken when turning an injured diver from the supine into the recovery position or onto the side. Avoid excessive movement and remember to protect the head, neck and spine.

Overview of Dive Accident Management

First priority always goes to airway, breathing and circulation *(ABCs)*.

Every injured diver in respiratory distress or whose injury suggests the possibility of hypoxia should receive oxygen as soon as it becomes available.

Every unresponsive injured diver should be assumed to have respiratory insufficiency and needs:

- Protection of airway;
- Careful monitoring to determine if rescue breathing is required;
- The highest possible concentration of inspired oxygen.

Airway, Breathing and Circulation (ABCs) are always the first priority when assisting an injured diver.

Remember, when in doubt, provide oxygen. Oxygen should never be withheld for any reason from anyone suspected of hypoxia.

When providing oxygen, check:

- Oxygen supply frequently;
- Adequate delivery of oxygen:
  - *Can you hear the demand valve opening?*
  - *Is the reservoir bag inflating and deflating?*
  - *Can you hear the flow of oxygen to the pocket mask?*
- The injured diver's condition.

Oxygen should never be withheld for any reason from anyone suspected of hypoxia.

Providing Oxygen for Divers

Upon completion of this course, you may have uncertainties about your ability to perform in a real situation. When someone is injured, anxiety is a natural reaction both for the injured diver and rescuers. You can expect to have a pounding heart and breathless feeling if you are suddenly confronted with an emergency of any kind. These feelings generally do not interfere with your ability to use your skills, and in fact, your knowledge and training should reduce the level of your anxiety.

There are other concerns, including the fear of making a mistake, harming an injured diver, or the possibility of death. Although unlikely, these concerns are real. However, it is more important to make the effort, since the person who needs assistance may be in worse shape without your help than with a possibly imperfect effort to provide assistance.

Rescuers may have another concern about liability and the possibility of being sued. Anyone can be sued for anything. However, if you act in good faith, as a reasonably prudent person would do, and perform appropriately within your realm of training and expertise, you have little fear of liability. Although an injured diver may not improve, this is not evidence that you were responsible or that you performed below standards.

Your responsibility as a first aid provider is to treat the injured diver, family, and friends with respect during an emotionally difficult situation. You should act in a decisive manner and perform according to your knowledge and skill level. You should also see that the injured diver is referred to medical care or to someone whose ability is equal to or greater than yours. You are not obligated to start a first aid procedure, but once you do, you must continue until you are relieved by someone with equal or greater skill and/or qualifications.

Although you are not obligated to start a first aid procedure, once you do, you must continue until you are relieved by someone with equal or greater skill.

Finally, practice what you have learned at every opportunity so that you will be prepared if your skills are needed.

Place the injured diver in the recommended position for dive accidents. If an injured diver vomits, temporarily discontinue oxygen use. After vomiting has ceased, evaluate the airway, clear if necessary and resume providing oxygen at the earliest possible moment.

Provide injured breathing divers with the highest possible concentration of oxygen by demand inhalator valve or non-rebreather mask. Adjust the flow rate to the non-rebreather mask so that the reservoir bag does not completely deflate during inhalations. If the reservoir bag is continually inflated, check the seal of the mask and adjust the flow rate accordingly.

Continue oxygen use until the injured diver has reached a definitive care facility or until the oxygen supply is depleted. Do not reduce oxygen flow to the injured diver in order to make the supply last. High concentrations of inhaled oxygen, even if delivered over a shorter period of time, will be more beneficial to the injured diver by creating a higher pressure gradient that results in a more effective washout of nitrogen.

Lower concentrations of inspired oxygen may not be as effective, even though the rescuer may be able to deliver oxygen for a longer period of time.

If the injured diver has a seizure, it may be necessary to remove the oxygen in order to evaluate the ABCs. Resume oxygen delivery as soon as possible after seizure ceases and the ABCs have been assessed.

Remember to frequently practice all first aid, resuscitation, CPR and related oxygen skills

Seizures occurring during surface oxygen administration are usually the result of a hypoxic event to the brain. Except to call for assistance with an unresponsive diver, never leave an injured diver alone or unattended while emergency oxygen is being provided.

A flow rate of 15 lpm is suggested for injured divers using constant flow with the non-rebreather mask or pocket mask.

Oral administration of fluids is recommended for the alert and oriented injured diver who is not at risk of vomiting. If oral fluids are given to the injured diver, water is recommended as it is rapidly absorbed by the body, and it presents a lower risk of inducing vomiting. Other non-carbonated, non-caffeinated beverages are acceptable if water is unavailable.

Remember to frequently practice all first aid, resuscitation, CPR and related oxygen skills.

Oxygen Safety Reminders

- Use oxygen only in well-ventilated areas.
- Extinguish all burning materials before oxygen is used.
- Never combine oxygen and flammables, like petroleum products. The combination of these materials may support spontaneous combustion in the presence of high-pressure oxygen.

Dive Accident Solution

Throughout this manual, you have reviewed several factors that may contribute to the dive accident problem. Now that you are informed as oxygen first aid providers, you are part of the dive accident solution.

As a prepared diver, you can do this by being able to recognize signs and symptoms of scuba diving injuries and illnesses.

Prepare a comprehensive Emergency Assistance Plan with a back-up. This includes having and knowing how to utilize communications equipment, the location of the nearest medical facility, and how to access the DAN 24-hour emergency hotline for medical consultation and assistance in locating an appropriate hyperbaric facility and assisting in transportation.

Activate the local Emergency Medical Services *(EMS)* if possible.

Have sufficient oxygen available until the injured diver arrives at the nearest available medical facility. Remember to avoid reducing the oxygen flow rate to the injured diver in order to make the supply last. Provide accident information to medical personnel.

Remember to go to the nearest, most appropriate medical facility and not necessarily to the nearest hyperbaric chamber. There are a number of reasons why an injured diver should be transported to the nearest hospital emergency department and not to the nearest recompression chamber:

- There are only a small number of hospitals equipped with hyperbaric chambers.
- Many hospitals with hyperbaric chambers are not equipped to treat diving injuries 24 hours a day. It takes time to assemble a chamber crew for a diving injury treatment.
- Many hospitals require a DAN or physician referral before accepting the transfer of an injured diver.
- Some chambers are open only when they have patients and are closed the rest of the time.
- Some chambers are not equipped to treat divers.
- Hyperbaric chamber status continually changes, and it is nearly impossible for any individual to maintain accurate daily information. This situation may create unnecessary delays if a dive team relies on obsolete information.
- DAN and most training agencies consider the practice of dive instructors advising students to go directly to the nearest chamber unwise.
- DAN advises divers to call the DAN or DAN-supported emergency number for your area, day or night, if you suspect a diving injury.
- Every dive injury is unique, and crucial medical decisions must be made individually by a physician trained in diving medicine. The decision on where to treat an injured diver can only be made after a thorough medical evaluation and appropriate consultation.

Transport an injured diver to the nearest hospital emergency department and not the nearest recompression chamber.

The first steps in an emergency are most critical in determining how the injured diver will recover:

- Remember S-A-V-E *(Stop, Assess scene, Ventilation for oxygen adequate, and Exposure protection).*
- Airway, Breathing, Circulation *(ABCs).*
- Provide 100 percent inspired oxygen.
- Contact the EMS and transport the injured diver to the nearest hospital emergency department.
- Call DAN or a DAN supported hotline for consultation.

Understand legal considerations:

- There are no medical contraindications for providing oxygen to an injured scuba diver. International laws are not well-defined for oxygen use and oxygen cylinder filling.

Understand misconceptions about oxygen and its use, and continue your education by reading up-to-date literature, taking other courses and learning from others.

Review Questions

1. Oxygen units should remain in a waterproof case, assembled and unpressurized.

a. True b. False

2. Oxygen cylinders should remain full and be refilled after each use.

a. True b. False

3. Oxygen units should be serviced every _______.

a. Year
b. Five years
c. Two years
d. Oxygen units do not need servicing.

4. Oxygen units and masks should be cleaned after each use.

a. True b. False

5. Match the following: The injured diver should be placed in which position?

Recovery Position ______
Supine Position ______
Position of Comfort ______

a. Responsive breathing diver
b. Unresponsive breathing diver
c. Unresponsive non-breathing injured diver

6. Injured divers should never be given any oral fluids.

a. True b. False

7. Injured divers should always be immediately transported to the nearest hyperbaric chamber.

a. True b. False

Answers

1. a
2. a
3. c
4. a
5. b, c, a
6. b
7. b

Glossary

Alveoli — Microscopic air sacs in the lungs where gas exchange occurs with the circulatory system.

Anoxia — Absence of oxygen in the circulating blood or in the tissues.

Aorta — The largest vessel of the systemic arterial system, from which the main arteries carrying oxygenated blood branch and subdivide into smaller and smaller vessels.

***Arterial Gas Embolism* (AGE)** — Gas bubbles in the arterial system generally caused by air passing through the walls of the alveoli into the bloodstream.

Arteriole — Small artery.

Atrium — Chamber of the heart which provides access to another chamber called the ventricle.

Bronchi — Plural of bronchus, which is a division of the trachea.

Bronchiole — Small branch of the bronchus that carries air to and from the alveoli.

Bronchospasm — Bronchoconstriction, or the sudden narrowing of the smaller airways, of a spasmodic nature.

Capillary — Microscopic blood vessels where the gas exchange takes place between the bloodstream and the tissues or the air in the lungs.

Carbon Dioxide — A waste gas produced by the metabolism of oxygen in the body.

Carbon Monoxide — A highly poisonous, odorless, tasteless and colorless gas formed when carbon material burns with restricted access to oxygen. It is toxic by inhalation since it competes with oxygen in binding with the hemoglobin, thereby resulting in diminished availability of oxygen in tissues.

Cartilaginous — Pertaining to or composed of cartilage.

Cilia — Long, slender microscopic hairlike processes extending from cells and capable of rhythmic motion.

CPR — Cardiopulmonary resuscitation.

***Decompression Illness* (DCI)** — Dysbaric injuries related to scuba diving, which includes both decompression sickness *(DCS)* and arterial gas embolism *(AGE).*

***Decompression Sickness* (DCS)** — A syndrome caused by bubbles of inert gas forming in the tissues and bloodstream which can evolve from too rapid an ascent from compressed gas diving.

Dehydration — An abnormal depletion of water and other body fluids.

***Diameter Indexing Safety System* (DISS)** — Intermediate pressure port where a hose attaches, leading to demand valve or other apparatus.

EMS — Emergency Medical Services

Epiglottis — Thin structure behind the tongue that shields the entrance of the larynx during swallowing, preventing the aspiration of debris into the trachea and lungs.

Erythroprotein — A protein which is synthesized mainly in the kidneys and stimulates red blood cell formation.

Esophagus — Portion of the digestive tract that lies between the back of the throat and stomach.

Fossa Ovalis — Oval depression in the wall of the heart remaining when the foramen ovale closes at birth *(See patent foramen ovale).*

Gradient — The difference in pressure, oxygen tension, or other variable as a function of distance, time or other continuously changing influence.

Hypoxemia — Inadequate oxygen supply in the arterial blood.

Hypoxia — Inadequate oxygen supply to the body tissues.

Inert — Having little or no tendency to react chemically.

Incontinence — Absence of voluntary control of an excretory function, especially defecation or urination.

Intercostal Muscles — The muscles between the ribs which contract during inspiration to increase the volume of the chest cavity.

Ischemia — Inadequate blood flow to a part or organ.

Larynx — The organ of voice production, also known as the voice box; the opening from the back of the throat into the trachea *(windpipe)*.

Laryngospasm — Severe constriction of the larynx in response to the introduction to water, allergies, or noxious stimuli.

LPM — Liters per minute. A measurement of a flow rate of gas or liquid.

Mediastinum — The space within the chest located between the lungs, that contains the heart, major blood vessels, trachea and esophagus.

Metabolism — The conversion of food into energy and waste products.

Nystagmus — Spontaneous, rapid, rhythmic movement of the eyes occurring on fixation or on ocular movement.

Oblique — An indirect or evasive angle.

Oxygen — A colorless, odorless, tasteless gas essential to life making up approximately 21 percent of air.

Occlude — To close off or stop up; obstruct.

Patent Foramen Ovale — A hole in the septum *(wall)* between the right and left atria of the heart.

Pericardium — A double-layered membranous sac surrounding the heart and major blood vessels connected to it.

Pharynx — Portion of the airway at the back of the throat, connecting mouth, nasal cavity and larynx.

Platelet — A round or oval disk found in the blood of vertebrate animals that are involved with blood clotting.

Pleura - Membranes surrounding the outer surface of the lungs and the inner surface of the chest wall and the diaphragm.

Prescription — A written order for dispensing drugs signed by a physician.

Primary Assessment — Assessment of the Airway, Breathing and Circulation *(pulse)* in an ill or injured person; also known as the ABCs.

PSI — Pounds per square inch; a measurement of pressure.

Respiration — The exchange of gases between a living organism and its environment; the act of breathing.

Respiratory Arrest — Cessation of breathing.

Sign — Any medical or trauma condition that can be observed and described.

Symptom — Any non-observable condition described by the patient.

Supine — Lying flat on back, with face upward.

Surfactant — A substance produced in the lungs to reduce surface tension in alveoli and small airways.

Thorax — The upper part of the trunk *(main part of the body)* between the neck and the abdomen which contains the heart, lungs, trachea and bronchi.

Trachea — The air passage that begins at the larynx and ends as the beginning of the principal right and left bronchi.

Valsalva Maneuver — The forced inflation of the middle ear by exhaling with the mouth closed and the nostrils pinched.

Venous Gas Emboli — Inert gas bubbles in venous blood (which return to the heart and lungs).

Ventricle — Thick-walled, muscular chamber in the heart which receives blood from the atrium, pumping it through to the pulmonary or systemic circulation.

Venules — Small veins.

Related Readings

American Red Cross. *Oxygen Administration.* St. Louis: Mosby-LifeLine, 1993.

American Red Cross. *Preventing Disease Transmission.* St. Louis: Mosby-LifeLine, 1993.

Anderson, L., and E. Atikkan. "Oxygen: Friend or Foe?" In *Proceedings of the 1992 IQ.* Montclair, Calif.: NAUI, 1992, pp. 1-3.

Baker, W., and A. Mossman, eds. Matheson Gas Data Book. *Matheson Gas Products.* 1971, pp. 441-445.

Bassett, B. "Oxygen: Is it a Miracle Drug for Divers." *Ocean Realm* (Fall 1986): 13-16.

Bennett, P., and D. Elliott. *The Physiology and Medicine of Diving.* 4th ed. London: W.B. Saunders, 1993.

Bertsch, J., and D. Orr. "Oxygen First Aid in Dive Accidents." *Alert Diver* (September/October 1991): 7.

Bookspan, J. "Is Oxygen a 'Feel Good' Gas for Divers?" *Underwater USA* (October 1992): 35.

Bove, A., and J. Davis. *Diving Medicine.* 2nd ed. Philadelphia:W.B. Saunders, 1990.

Bove, F. "Diving Medicine: Oxygen." *Skin Diver* (June 1985): 16.

Bozanic, J. "Diver's Forum: Should Instructors be Required to Have Oxygen Administration Equipment and Training to Maintain in Teaching Status?" *Sources* (May/June 1990): 9-12.

Bunting, K., and K. Shoenberger. "Administering Oxygen: What You Need to Know." *Nursing 90,* no. 20 (June 1990): 47-51.

Clendenen, W. "The Four R's of Managing a DCI Injury." *Alert Diver* (January/February 1996): 26-29.

Clendenen, W. "The Pocket Mask." *Alert Diver* (November/December 1996): 32-36.

Clendenen, W. "Your Dive Education." *Alert Diver* (November/December 1995): 34-39.

Compressed Gas Association Inc. "Characteristics and Safe Handling of Medical Gases." Arlington, Va.: CGA, P-2.

Compressed Gas Association Inc. "Cleaning Equipment for Oxygen Service." Arlington, Va.: CGA, G-4.1.

Compressed Gas Association Inc. "Commodity Specification for Oxygen." Arlington, Va.: CGA, G-4.3.

Compressed Gas Association Inc. "Filling of Industrial and Medical Nonflammable Compressed Gas Cylinders." Arlington, Va.: CGA, P-15.

Compressed Gas Association Inc. "Handbook of Compressed Gases." 3rd ed., Arlington, Va.: CGA.

Compressed Gas Association Inc. "Oxygen." Arlington, Va.: CGA, G-4.

Compressed Gas Association Inc. "Safe Handling of Compressed Gases in Containers." Arlington, Va.: CGA, P-1.

Corry, J. "The Importance of O2 Treatment And Training." *NAUI News* (November/December 1988): 44-46.

Corry, J. "Oxygen Administration Course Available." *Underwater USA* (January 1989): 35.

Corry, J. "Oxygen Training — Needed and Available." *NAUI News* (September/October 1988): 41, 43.

Corry, J. "Setting the Record Straight: Oxygen Delivery and the Injured Diver." In *Diving Accident Management,* ed. P. Bennett and R. Moon, 323-342. Bethesda, Md.: UHMS, 1990.

Corry, J. "Setting the Record Straight: Oxygen Delivery and the Injured Diver." In *IQ 1991 Proceedings,* ed. H. Viders and F. Wells, 29-44. Montclair, Calif.: NAUI, 1991.

Corry, J. *Student Workbook for Emergency Oxygen Administration and Field Management of Scuba Diving Accidents Workshop.* Montclair, Calif.: NAUI, 1987, 77 pages.

Corry, J. *Student Workbook for Emergency Oxygen Administration.* Montclair, Calif.: NAUI, 1989.

Corry, J. "Unique Oxygen Training Course Developed by Diving Community." *Response* (Winter 1990): 17-18. Also. *Alert Diver* 4, no. 2 (Summer 1988): 10.

Davis, J., and T. Hunt, eds. *Hyberbaric Oxygen Therapy.* Bethesda, Md.: UMS, 1977.

Dick, A., P. Bennett, and J. Miller. "Oxygen & Diving Accidents." *Undersea Journal* (Third Quarter 1983): 23.

Dick, A., P. Bennett, and J. Miller. "Oxygen And Scuba Diving Accidents." *Scuba Times* (May/June 1983): 26-27; Also: *Alert Diver* 2, no. 1 (Spring 1985): 1-2.

Donald, K. *Oxygen and the Diver.* Self-Publishing, Great Britain: Hanley Swan, 1992, 256 pages

Dovenbarger, J. "Oxygen Use in Dive Accidents." *Alert Diver* 4, no. 2 (Summer 1988): 12-13.

Dovenbarger, J. *DAN Report on Diving Accidents and Fatalities.* Durham, N.C.: Divers Alert Network, 1987-1997 annual.

Edmonds, C., C. Lowry, and J. Pennefather. *Diving and Subaquatic Medicine.* 3rd ed. Oxford, England: Butterworth-Heinemann, 1992.

Edmonds, C., B. McKenzie, and R. Thomas. *Diving Medicine for Scuba Divers.* 1992.

Elling, R. "An Evaluation of Emergency Medical Technician's Ability to Use Manual Ventilation Devices." *Ann. Emerg. Med.* 12, no. 12 (December 1983): 765-768.

Gorman, D. "Decompression Sickness and Arterial Gas Embolism in Sports Scuba Divers." *Sports Medicine* 8, no. 1 (1989): 32-42.

Greer, H., and E. Massey. "Neurologic Injury From Undersea Diving." *Neurologic Clinics* 10, no. 4 (1992): 1031-1045.

Hardy, J. "The Role of Oxygen in Diving Emergencies." *Diver* (February 1985): 8-9.

Harpour, G. "The Role of Oxygen in Diving Emergencies." *Canadian Diving Journal,* no. 2 (1985): 20-21.

Hendrick, W., and B. Thomson. *Oxygen and the Scuba Diver.* Hurley, N.Y.: Lifeguard Systems, 1988.

Howard, P. *Oxygen Therapy.* Wright, England: Bristol Publishing, 1987.

Hunt, J., and W. Clendenen. "Mind and Body." *Alert Diver* (July/August 1995): 30-35.

Jain, K., and B. Fischer. *Oxygen in Physiology and Medicine.* Springfield, Ill.: C.C. Thomas, 1989.

Jerrard, D. "Diving Medicine." *Emergency Medicine Clinics of North America* 10, no. 2, pp. 329-338.

Johannigman, J., and R. Branson. "Oxygen Enrichment of Expired Gas for Mouth-to-Mask Resuscitation." *Respiratory Care* 36, no. 2 (February 1991): 99-103.

Kindwall, E., ed. *Hyperbaric Medicine Practice.* Flagstaff, Ariz.: Best Publishing Co., 1995.

Kindwall, E. "Oxygen Fire Caused by Quick Opening Ball Valve" *Pressure* 21, no. 2 (March/April 1992): 10.

Kizer, K. "Delayed Treatment of Dysbarism." *JAMA* 247, no. 18 (1982): 2555-2558.

Lambertsen, C., G. Bond, and J. Jacobson, ed. "Hyperbaric Oxygenation." *Annals of the New York Academy of Sciences* 117, no. 2, pp. 647-890.

Larrymore, M. "Fire Hazards in Oxygen Systems Covered by ASTM." *Pressure* (July/August 1992): 7-8; Part 2: (November/December 1992): 5.

Lippmann, J., and S. Bugg. *The DAN Emergency Handbook.* 3rd ed. Carnegie, Australia: J.L. Publications, 1995.

Lippmann, J. *Deeper into Diving.* Locust Valley, N.Y.: Aqua Quest Publications, 1990, pp. 499-521.

Lippmann, J. "Oxygen First Aid." *Undersea Journal* (3rd Quarter 1994): 55-59.

Lippmann, J. *Oxygen First Aid for Divers.* Carnegie, Australia: J. L. Publications, Australia: 1992, US: 1992.

Lippmann, J., and S. Bugg. "Oxygen Treatment." *Alert Diver* (February/March 1990): 22.

Loewenherz, J. "Pathophysiology and Treatment of Decompression Sickness and Gas Embolism." *J. Florida M.A.* 79, no. 9 (1992): 620-624.

Mebane, G.Y., ed. *DAN Dive and Travel Medical Guide.* Durham, N.C.: Divers Alert Network, 1995.

Miles, S., and D. MacKay. *Underwater Medicine* London: Granada Publishing (1976): 95-116.

Motesso. V., et al. "Comparison of Delivered Volumes and Airway Pressures When Ventilating Through an Endotracheal Tube With Bag-Valve vs. Demand-Valve." *Prehospital & Disaster Medicine* 9, no. 1 (January/March 1994): 24-27.

Mount, T. "Oxygen Management." *Sport Diver* (July/August 1994): 20-23.

National Fire Protection Association. "Fire Hazards in Oxygen-Enriched Atmospheres." *NFPA Manual,* Quincy, Mass., 53M-1990.

National Research Council. *Fundamentals of Hyperbaric Medicine.* Washington, D.C.: Committee on Hyperbaric Medicine, NRC, 1966.

NOAA, *NOAA Diving Manual,* 1991.

Orr, D. "Incident Insights — Doing the Right Thing." *Alert Diver* (November/December 1995): 21.

Orr, D. "Incident Insights — Diver, Don't Heal Thyself." *Alert Diver* (September/October 1995): 21.

Orr, D., and J. Bertsch. "Divers Alert Network (DAN) Oxygen First Aid in Dive Accidents." *Street Skills Magazine* (1995).

Pierce, A. "A Smoldering Spark of Life." In *IQ 14 Proceedings,* ed. B. Bridge, 180-185. Montclair, Calif.: NAUI, 1983.

Porter, C. "Instructor Attitudes on Carrying Oxygen." *NAUI News* (January/February 1989): 40-41.

Rioux, T. "Oxygen Capability for Small Wet Boats." In *Coldwater Diving for Science, 1987,* ed. M. Lang, 205-231. Costa Mesa, Calif.: AAUS, 1987.

Rutledge, R. "Oxygen Delivery Systems." In *IQ 14 Proceedings,* ed. B. Bridge, 199-203. Montclair, Calif.: NAUI, 1983.

Rutledge, R. "Oxygen Delivery Systems." *NAUI News* (November 1984): 17-19.

Ryan, R. "Hyperbaric Oxygen Therapy for Diving Casualties." In *Proceedings of the 1992 IQ,* 181-186. Montclair, Calif.: NAUI, 1992.

Schilling, C., and M. Faiman. "Physics of Diving and Physical Effects on Divers." In *The Physician's Guide to Diving Medicine,* ed. C. Schilling, C. Carston, and R. Mathias, 39-41. New York, N.Y.: Plenum Press, 1984.

Stone, T. "Oxygen and Diving." *Discover Diving* (March/April 1992): 10-11.

Sweeney, L. "Can You Legally Give Oxygen to a Diving Accident Victim in Your State?" *Underwater USA* (May 1990): 36.

Sweeney, L. "Doctor Invents Emergency O2 Device." *Underwater USA* (October 1992): 14-15.

Taylor, L. "A Diver's Guide to Oxygen Therapy Apparatus." *Sources* Part 1: (July/August 1989): 30-35; Part 2: (September/October 1989): 72-74.

Taylor, L. "A Higher Concentration Oxygen Delivery Pocket Mask." *NAUI News* (March/April 1989): 40. Also: *Alert Diver* 5, no. 3 (Fall 1989): 15.

Taylor, L. "Rx: Oxygen." *NAUI News* (November/December 1986): 28-29. Also: *Alert Diver* 2, no. 5 (Summer 1986): 10.

Trimble, V. *The Uncertain Miracle.* Garden City, N.Y.: Doubleday, 1974, 233 pages.

USDOT. *EMT-Basic National Standard Curriculum.* NHTSA, 1994.

USN. *US Navy Divers Handbook.* Revised 1993.

Vann, R. "The Oxygen Window." *Alert Diver* (January/February 1993): 14-16.

Viders, H. "Emergency Oxygen Administration: A New Device May Solve an Old Dispute." *Sources* (January/February 1995): 28-29.

Viders, H. "Emergency Oxygen: How Much Is Enough?" *Scuba Times* (November/December 1992): 22-23.

Viders, H. "Emergency Oxygen: Which Equipment Is Best?" *Scuba Times* (September/October 1993): 48-50.

Weiss, L., and K. Van Meter. "The Application of Hyperbaric Oxygen Therapy in Emergency Medicine." *Am. J. Emer. Med.* 10, no. 6 (1992): 558-568.

Wells, F. "Report on State Laws and Regulations Concerning the Use and Dispensing of Oxygen by Providers of First Aid." Document furnished to NAUI by author, 1989.

Zaferes, A. "Oxygen Administration, Is It for You?" *Sources* (July/August 1990): 51, 56.

Notes

Notes